APHASIOLOGY

APHASIOLOGY is covered by the following abstracting and indexing services: *BLLDB (Bibliography of Linguistic Literature), CINAHL, Current Contents, Elsevier Science BV, EMBASE/Excerpta Medica, Linguistic Abstracts, Linguistic and Language Behavior Abstracts, Medical Documentation Service, PsycINFO, PsycBITE, Research Alert, Science Citation Index, SciSearch, SCOPUS, UnCover.*

APHASIOLOGY

Volume 26 Number 9 September 2012

Special Issue: Brain stimulation and language

Guest Editor: Jenny Crinion

CONTENTS

First published 2012 by Psychology Press

Published 2018 by Routledge
2 Park Square, Milton Park, Abingdon, Oxon OX14 4RN
52 Vanderbilt Avenue, New York, NY 10017

First issued in hardback 2018

Routledge is an imprint of the Taylor & Francis Group, an informa business

Typeset by Integra Software Services Pvt. Ltd, India.

ISBN 13: 978-1-138-40390-1 (hbk)
ISBN 13: 978-1-84872-769-4 (pbk)

APHASIOLOGY, 2012, 26 (9), 1077–1081

EDITORIAL

Shocking speech

Jenny Crinion

Institute of Cognitive Neuroscience, University College London, London, UK

Over one million people in the United States and 250,000 people in the United Kingdom are living today with aphasia (Code & Petheram, 2011; Dickey et al., 2010). To put these numbers in context, it is more prevalent than, for example, Parkinson's disease and multiple sclerosis. Furthermore, as a result of stroke alone, 100,000 new patients are added to the total aphasia population each year from these two countries. Yet, in spite of its high incidence, aphasia is still a hidden disability, isolating patients and relatives. Aphasia therapy that is properly selected, carefully targeted to specific aphasic symptoms and administered with sufficient dosage does work (Bhogal, Teasell, & Foley, 2003; Cicerone et al., 2011; Code, 2012; Kelly, Brady, & Enderby, 2010). Most language interventions are administered by speech-language therapists who evaluate patients' individual needs, and then use a combination of face-to-face, group, and computer-delivered techniques tailored to the individual patient's impairment profile. Nevertheless, despite extensive behavioural therapy that can be costly and difficult to achieve with limited resources, recovery is frequently incomplete and frustratingly slow. Interestingly, half of elderly aphasic patients are unwilling to participate in intensive behavioural training, particularly if they have received therapy before, and still others initiate rehabilitation but abandon before the minimum period required for improvement (Basso & Macis, 2011). Improved rehabilitation methods are needed to achieve higher levels of recovery within a shorter time frame. This has led researchers to consider complementary brain stimulating strategies to treat aphasia such as drugs (Berthier, Pulvermuller, Davila, Casares, & Butierrez, 2011) and non-invasive transcranial electrical or magnetic brain stimulation techniques or invasive epidural cortical stimulation. This special issue of *Aphasiology* reviews the exciting new field of neuromodulation using these cortical stimulation techniques to enhance recovery and supplement the effects of aphasia rehabilitation.

Several forms of brain stimulation have been examined as a means to change brain function and thereby promote neuroplasticity (Plow, Carey, Nudo, & Pascual-Leone, 2009; Webster, Celnik, & Cohen, 2006). At the present time most studies of non-invasive brain stimulation have been conducted in healthy volunteers, proving the properties of these techniques that induce long-lasting, changes on neural excitability within specific brain areas, see Flöel (2012) for a review of language

Address correspondence to: Jenny Crinion, MRC Clinical Scientist, Institute of Cognitive Neuroscience, University College London, 17 Queen Square, London, WC1N 3AR, UK. E-mail: j.crinion@ucl.ac.uk

http://dx.doi.org/10.1080/02687038.2012.714215

studies. Chief among these used in stroke rehabilitation include repetitive transcranial magnetic stimulation (rTMS) and anodal or cathodal transcranial direct current stimulation (tDCS), delivered to the ipsilesional, or contralesional hemisphere. The aims being to either increase ipsilesional excitability or decrease contralesional excitability. The small number of aphasia studies that have applied TMS or tDCS to investigate its therapeutic effects—primarily on speech production—have obtained mixed, albeit mostly positive, results. Using these non-invasive methods in clinical practice could bring enormous gains for the treatment of aphasia. However, particular focus in clinical trials is on tDCS as it is portable, non-expensive, safe (lower risk of seizures than TMS) and involves a relatively simple set-up. These features make tDCS a putative candidate for home treatment as an add-on to behavioural training or substitutive therapy for pharmacological treatments. In this special issue we consider the role of both invasive (Cherney et al., 2012) and non-invasive brain stimulation (Holland & Crinion, 2012; Medina et al., 2012) in the treatment of post-stroke aphasia, the evidence for efficacy of different methods (Flöel, 2012; Hoffman, Pobric, Drakesmith, & Lambon Ralph, 2012; Möttönen & Watkins, 2012), and the theory-based explanations of stimulation-related benefits for aphasia recovery and rehabilitation (Hartwigsen & Siebner, 2012).

At present there are no universally accepted methods or "gold standards" for the treatment of aphasia against which these new or experimental interventions can be compared. Nevertheless, most therapists, clinicians, and researchers in the aphasia field would agree that a treatment should be considered clinically meaningful and effective if (1) patients show significant improvement in trained compared to untrained items; (2) that these behavioural effects persist beyond the training period; and (3) that any improvement in impairment-based measures generalises to real-world contexts. For example, a patient's improvement in spoken picture naming is accompanied with improvement in their functional communication skills as they apply their renewed vocabulary in daily life. This is an important concept to keep in mind when discussing the various brain stimulation studies that have been conducted so far and highlighted in this special issue. Following stroke the functional improvement from non-invasive brain stimulation methods alone is reported to be only 10% to 30% and is short-lasting (Hummel & Cohen, 2006; Talelli & Rothwell, 2006; Webster et al., 2006). In the search for more effective and longer-lasting interventions, the combination of rehabilitation and brain stimulation seems reasonable. Indeed animal studies have shown that the combination of peripheral and central stimulation enhances synaptic plasticity more than central stimulation alone (Fritsch et al., 2010). Brain stimulation, not as a complete therapy in itself but as an adjunct to other therapies, may magnify therapeutic outcomes.

A key question relates to timing. Should brain stimulation methods be applied before, during, or after a behavioural therapy? In this context the impact of the type of behavioural coupling with stimulation needs to be carefully considered. Fluctuations in brain activity before or after stimulation can impact the effect of cortical stimulation. Homeostatic plasticity, as conceptualised by the Binenstock-Cooper-Monroe theory (Bienenstock, Cooper, & Munro, 1982) proposes that learning, through long-term potentiation-inducing mechanisms, strengthens synaptic connections to a level such that the effect of a subsequent long-term potentiation-inducing protocol is occluded (Ziemann, Ilic, Pauli, Meintzschel, & Ruge, 2004). Thus the specific timing between rehabilitation and cortical stimulation is critical. Additionally, state-dependency, i.e., a targeted region's varying response to stimulation based on its previous state of activity, should be studied in the context of combination of rehabilitation with stimulation (Silvanto, Cattaneo, Battelli, & Pascual-Leone, 2008). If the desired effect is enhancing task performance, then it may be ideal to stimulate before or during therapy, in order to prime particular brain areas. A number of tDCS studies have reported positive effects on language task performance during stimulation (see Flöel [2012], and Holland & Crinion [2012] for reviews of studies in healthy and aphasic participants respectively). However, if the desired effect is on consolidation, then it may be best to apply the stimulation either during or after therapy. A recent proof-of-concept study showed that a combination of an intonation-based therapy and simultaneous anodal tDCS over the right inferior frontal gyrus (IFG) led to an improvement in speech fluency compared to a condition in which sham tDCS was applied to aphasic patients receiving intonation-based therapy (Vines, Norton, & Schlaug, 2011). In the context of neuro-rehabilitation of aphasia, applying stimulation during aphasia therapy has the potential to influence both the immediate language performance and the consolidation phases of relearning.

Customising non-invasive stimulation to the neural activation is also likely to be important. A focal stimulation by means of TMS does not only alter connectivity of the brain region stimulated, but also of areas distant to the stimulation site (Bestmann, Baudewig, Siebner, Rothwell, & Frahm, 2005). This implies that behavioural effects evolving after stimulation are based on a remodelling of the whole neural network rather than being caused by excitability changes of a single brain region. Stroke and other neurological diseases typically affect complex behaviours like speech, by disrupting large-scale neural systems, hence a network approach is likely to be better suited to investigate the pathophysiology underlying neurological deficits in the damaged brain than conventional functional MRI studies. To address this, in this special issue of *Aphasiology* three studies (Hartwigsen & Siebner, 2012; Hoffman et al., 2012; Möttönen & Watkins, 2012) employed transcranial magnetic stimulation (TMS) to offer important insights into the causality of neural connectivity. Functional imaging studies are useful in revealing brain regions that patients activate during language tasks, however, they do not provide information about causality. Accordingly, areas that are active during task performance may not be functionally critical but merely a secondary effect. For example, to examine whether right hemisphere activation in aphasia are correlating with the recovery process, recent studies have focused on facilitating the left or inhibiting the right IFG, particularly the triangular portion, to test whether short term improvements in language can be observed (Baker, Rorden, & Fridriksson, 2010; Fridriksson, Richardson, Baker, & Rorden, 2011; Weiduschat et al., 2011). In addition several reports (Vines et al., 2011), including one featured in this special issue (Medina et al., 2012) have described therapies that specifically engage or stimulate the homologous right hemisphere regions, which might have the potential to facilitate the language recovery process beyond the limitations of natural recovery.

Can a patient's genetic make-up influence their responsiveness to brain stimulation? Most of the work done to address this has been in treatment of limb function following stroke. For example, Malcolm et al. (2007), in a study of rTMS of the affected hemisphere, found a subgroup of patients showing desirable effects from stimulation ("stimulation responders"). "Stimulation responsiveness" could be a consequence of genetic predispositions. Indeed, it has been found that "absence of val66met polymorphism" in the brain-derived neurotrophic factor (BDNF) gene allows for training induced cortical reorganisation in human motor cortex (Kleim et al., 2006). Furthermore, "stimulation responsiveness" could also be artificially promoted by customising cortical stimulation to the cortical activation and function of patients. Nowak et al. (2008) treated patients who showed contralesional recruitment of the dorsal premotor cortex in association with poor baseline limb function by using inhibitory 1 Hz rTMS over the contralesional M1. More recently Witte et al. (2012) showed that genotype-related differences in neurophysiology (BDNF x catechol-O-methyltransferase interaction) translated into behavioural differences for implicit grammar and motor learning. These findings might contribute to a better understanding of the mechanisms of inter-individual differences in learning or aphasic patients' relearning. Thus, to predict the stimulation responsiveness, use of neurophysiological mapping or functional neuroimaging may be critical at least in this early stage of application to aphasia rehabilitation.

Brain stimulation interventions modulating stroke-induced disruption of diverse neural networks may improve language and communication deficits in aphasic patients through facilitation of brain plasticity and long-term potentiation. Benefits are not evident for all methods and refinement in clinical trial designs is required. Preliminary data suggests that combining stimulation and behavioural training are associated with better outcomes than other strategies and long-term maintenance of benefits. Some brain stimulation trials have failed because stimulation was not combined with speech and language therapy while other trials combining brain stimulation with model-driven therapies also probably failed because of short-trial duration, inadequate sample selection, or lack of stimulation effects. Lessons from non-invasive brain stimulation trials about task specificity and participant selection should also be understood to plan more valid designs in the future. Although further studies are needed, the current state of the evidence as outlined in this special issue of *Aphasiology* suggests that brain stimulation may play an exciting and key role in the treatment of post-stroke aphasia. It is a stimulating topic!

REFERENCES

Baker, J. M., Rorden, C., & Fridriksson, J. (2010). Using transcranial direct-current stimulation to treat stroke patients with aphasia. *Stroke*, *41*, 1229–1236.

Basso, A., & Macis, M. (2011). Therapy efficacy in chronic aphasia. *Behavioural Neurology*, *24*, 317–325.

Berthier, M. L., Pulvermuller, F., Davila, G., Casares, N. G., & Gutierrez, A. (2011). Drug therapy of post-stroke aphasia: a review of current evidence. *Neuropsychology Review*, *21*, 302–317.

Bestmann, S., Baudewig, J., Siebner, H. R., Rothwell, J. C., & Frahm, J. (2005). BOLD MRI responses to repetitive TMS over human dorsal premotor cortex. *Neuroimage*, *28*, 22–29.

Bhogal, S. K., Teasell, R. W., Foley, N. C., & Speechley, M. R. (2003). Rehabilitation of aphasia: More is better. *Topics in Stroke Rehabilitation*, *10*, 66–76.

Bienenstock, E. L., Cooper, L. N., & Munro, P. W. (1982). Theory for the development of neuron selectivity: Orientation specificity and binocular interaction in visual cortex. *The Journal of Neuroscience*, *2*, 32–48.

Cherney, L. R., Harvey, R. L., Babbitt, E. M., Hurwitz, R., Kaye, R. C., Lee, J. B., & Small, S. L. (2012). Epidural cortical stimulation and aphasia therapy. *Aphasiology*, *26*, 1192–1217.

Cicerone, K. D., Langenbahn, D. M., Braden, C., Malec, J. F., Kalmar, K., Fraas, M., . . . Ashman, T. (2011). Evidence-based cognitive rehabilitation: Updated review of the literature from 2003 through 2008. *Archives of Physical Medicine and Rehabilitation*, *92*, 519–530.

Code, C. (2012). Apportioning time for aphasia rehabilitation. *Aphasiology*, *26*, 729–735.

Code, C., & Petheram, B. (2011). Delivering for aphasia. *International Journal of Speech-Language Pathology*, *13*, 3–10.

Dickey, L., Kagan, A., Lindsay, M. P., Fang, J., Rowland, A., & Black, S. (2010). Incidence and profile of inpatient stroke-induced aphasia in Ontario, Canada. *Archives of Physical Medicine and Rehabilitation*, *91*, 196–202.

Flöel, A. (2012). Non-invasive brain stimulation and language processing in the healthy brain. *Aphasiology*, *26*, 1082–1102.

Fridriksson, J., Richardson, J. D., Baker, J. M., & Rorden, C. (2011). Transcranial direct current stimulation improves naming reaction time in fluent aphasia: A double-blind, sham-controlled study. *Stroke*, *42*, 819–821.

Fritsch, B., Reis, J., Martinowich, K., Schambra, H. M., Ji, Y., Cohen, L. G., & Lu, B. (2010). Direct current stimulation promotes BDNF-dependent synaptic plasticity: Potential implications for motor learning. *Neuron*, *66*, 198–204.

Hartwigsen, G., & Siebner, H. R. (2012). Probing the involvement of the right hemisphere in language processing with online transcranial magnetic stimulation in healthy volunteers. *Aphasiology*, *26*, 1131–1152.

Hoffman, P., Pobric, G., Drakesmith, M., & Lambon Ralph, M. A. (2012). Posterior middle temporal gyrus is involved in verbal and non-verbal semantic cognition: Evidence from rTMS. *Aphasiology*, *26*, 1119–1130.

Holland, R., & Crinion, J. (2012). Can tDCS enhance treatment of aphasia after stroke? *Aphasiology*, *26*, 1169–1191.

Hummel, F. C., & Cohen, L. G. (2006). Non-invasive brain stimulation: A new strategy to improve neurorehabilitation after stroke? *Lancet Neurology*, *5*, 708–712.

Kelly, H., Brady, M. C., & Enderby, P. (2010). Speech and language therapy for aphasia following stroke. *Cochrane Database of Systematic Reviews*, CD000425. DOI: 10.1002/14651858.CD000425.pub2

Kleim, J. A., Chan, S., Pringle, E., Schallert, K., Procaccio, V., Jimenez, R., & Cramer, S. C. (2006). BDNF val66met polymorphism is associated with modified experience-dependent plasticity in human motor cortex. *Nature Neuroscience*, *9*, 735–737.

Malcolm, M. P., Triggs, W. J., Light, K. E., Gonzalez Rothi, L. J., Wu, S., Reid, K., & Stephen, E. (2007). Repetitive transcranial magnetic stimulation as an adjunct to constraint-induced therapy: An exploratory randomized controlled trial. *American Journal of Physical Medicine & Rehabilitation/Association of Academic Physiatrists*, *86*, 707–715.

Medina, J., Norise, C., Faseyitan, O., Coslett, H. B., Turkeltaub, P. E., & Hamilton, R. H. (2012). Finding the right words: Transcranial magnetic stimulation improves discourse productivity in non-fluent aphasia after stroke. *Aphasiology*, *26*, 1153–1168.

Möttönen, R., & Watkins, K. E. (2012). Using TMS to study the role of the articulatory motor system in speech perception. *Aphasiology*, *26*, 1103–1118.

Nowak, D. A., Grefkes, C., Dafotakis, M., Eickhoff, S., Küst, J., Karbe, H., & Fink, G. R. (2008). Effects of low-frequency repetitive transcranial magnetic stimulation of the contralesional primary motor cortex on movement kinematics and neural activity in subcortical stroke. *Archives of Neurology*, *65*, 741–747.

Plow, E. B., Carey, J. R., Nudo, R. J., & Pascual-Leone, A. (2009). Invasive cortical stimulation to promote recovery of function after stroke: A critical appraisal. *Stroke*, *40*, 1926–1931.

Silvanto, J., Cattaneo, Z., Battelli, L., & Pascual-Leone, A. (2008). Baseline cortical excitability determines whether TMS disrupts or facilitates behavior. *Journal of Neurophysiology*, *99*, 2725–2730.

Talelli, P., & Rothwell, J. (2006). Does brain stimulation after stroke have a future? *Current Opinion in Neurology*, *19*, 543–550.

Vines, B. W., Norton, A. C., & Schlaug, G. (2011). Non-invasive brain stimulation enhances the effects of melodic intonation therapy. *Frontiers in Psychology*, *2*, 230.

Webster, B. R., Celnik, P. A., & Cohen, L. G. (2006). Non-invasive brain stimulation in stroke rehabilitation. *NeuroRx: The Journal of the American Society for Experimental NeuroTherapeutics*, *3*, 474–481.

Weiduschat, N., Thiel, A., Rubi-Fessen, I., Hartmann, A., Kessler, J., Merl, P., . . . Heiss, W. D. (2011). Effects of repetitive transcranial magnetic stimulation in aphasic stroke: A randomized controlled pilot study. *Stroke*, *42*, 409–415.

Witte, A. V., Kurten, J., Jansen, S., Schirmacher, A., Brand, E., Sommer, J., & Flöel, A. (2012). Interaction of BDNF and COMT polymorphisms on paired-associative stimulation-induced cortical plasticity. *The Journal of Neuroscience*, *32*, 4553–4561.

Ziemann, U., Ilic, T. V., Pauli, C., Meintzschel, F., & Ruge, D. (2004). Learning modifies subsequent induction of long-term potentiation-like and long-term depression-like plasticity in human motor cortex. *The Journal of Neuroscience*, *24*, 1666–1672.

APHASIOLOGY, 2012, 26 (9), 1082–1102

Non-invasive brain stimulation and language processing in the healthy brain

Agnes Flöel

Department of Neurology, Charite Universitätsmedizin Berlin, Center for Stroke Research Berlin, and Neurocure Cluster of Excellence Berlin, Germany

Background: Non-invasive brain stimulation (NIBS) has been used as a probe to modulate cognitive functions in humans for the last 20 years. The two most commonly reported techniques are transcranial magnetic stimulation (TMS) and transcranial direct current stimulation (tDCS), which have both been used with different stimulation parameters to increase or decrease excitability in target cortical regions.
Aims: In the present review, we highlight recent developments in TMS and tDCS in language research in healthy individuals.
Main Contribution: We will first describe how tDCS and TMS have been employed to improve either performance of language tasks, or learning in the language domain (facilitatory brain stimulation). Then, we will show how these techniques were used as interference techniques (inhibitory brain stimulation) for understanding brain–behaviour interactions and to explore possible cause–effect links between altered activity in specific brain areas and particular behaviours. We will only review studies in healthy individuals, and first pilot trials in patient population with more general cognitive impairments (idiopathic Parkinson's Disease, Alzheimer's Disease). For tDCS studies in aphasia, see Holland and Crinion (2012); for TMS studies in aphasia, see Medina et al. (2012).
Conclusions: In the healthy brain, NIBS can be used to delineate the functional significance of a particular brain region for the respective language task under study. Here, new possibilities of combining TMS or tDCS with functional imaging techniques offer unique opportunities to not only address the functional significance of a brain area underlying the coil or electrode, but in addition allow testing NIBS effects on an entire network. In this setting, TMS, both in its single-pulse and its repetitive form, allows the modulation of a specific function within milliseconds (single-pulse) or the order of seconds (particularly high-frequency rTMS trains), while tDCS has the disadvantage of requiring longer stimulation times. On the other hand, the relatively easy use of tDCS in the magnetic resonance scanner environment will render simultaneous recording of brain function and activation much more accessible, thus offering novel avenues in the study of network effects of NIBS. For proof-of principle studies to improve language learning in the healthy brain, tDCS may be the most fruitful approach due to its easy applicability and excellent safety profile. Subsequent use of this technique in parallel to training protocols to improve re-acquisition of language functions aphasic patients offers exciting possibilities in the realm of neurorehabilitation.

Address correspondence to: Agnes Flöel, Department of Neurology, Charite Universitätsmedizin Berlin, Center for Stroke Research Berlin, and Neurocure Cluster of Excellence Berlin, Chariteplatz 1, 10117 Berlin, Germany. E-mail: agnes.floeel@charite.de

http://dx.doi.org/10.1080/02687038.2011.589892

Keywords: Transcranial direct current stimulation; tDCS; Transcranial magnetic stimulation; TMS; Learning; Functional magnetic resonance imaging.

The basis for using brain stimulation in studies exploring the language system, as well as rehabilitation of aphasic deficits after stroke, is its potential to modulate cortical excitability and plasticity, and to facilitate the beneficial effects of training protocols. Two non-invasive brain stimulation (NIBS) techniques, transcranial magnetic stimulation (TMS) and transcranial direct current stimulation (tDCS), are currently being used. An invasive stimulation technique, epidural stimulation, is not of course used for studies in healthy individuals, but has been used in language rehabilitation; for more information, please see Cherney et al. in this special issue.

TMS is a NIBS technique based on Faraday's principle of electromagnetic induction. A brief pulse of current flowing through a coil of wire generates a magnetic field which, in turn, results in an electric field and currents that flow parallel to the plane of the coil (Rossini et al., 1994). Due to the electrical conductivity of living tissue the electric field leads to an electrical current in the cortex and subsequently to depolarisation of the underlying neurons (Hallett, 2007). Repetitive administration of < 1 Hz has been named low-frequency repetitive (r)TMS, and rTMS > 1 Hz as high-frequency rTMS. Transcranial direct current stimulation (tDCS) modulates cortical excitability by application of weak electrical currents in the form of direct current brain polarisation. Depending on direct current (DC) polarity, neuronal firing rates increase or decrease, presumably due to DC-induced changes in resting membrane potentials (Nitsche, Liebetanz, et al., 2003). The after-effects of tDCS on cortical excitability appear to be influenced by N-methyl-D-aspartate (NMDA) receptor-dependent processes (Nitsche, Jaussi, et al., 2004). High-frequency rTMS and anodal tDCS may increase motor-cortical excitability, while low-frequency rTMS and cathodal tDCS may decrease excitability (Chen et al., 1997; Hallett, 2007; Nitsche & Paulus, 2000, 2001). Furthermore, animal and human studies indicated that both techniques may influence long-term potentiation (LTP)-like and long-term depression (LTD)-like mechanisms, increase neurotrophic substances, dopamine and serotonine levels, and modulate gene expression ("immediate early genes") (Kuo, Paulus, & Nitsche, 2008; Liebetanz, Nitsche, Tergau, & Paulus, 2002; Nitsche, Grundey, et al., 2004; Nitsche et al., 2009; Strafella, Paus, Fraraccio, & Dagher, 2003). For epidural stimulation the exact mechanisms of action are not yet fully understood. Both facilitation of stimulated motor regions, similar to what has been shown for anodal tDCS or facilitatory rTMS, as well as inhibition of regions that have developed hyperactivity after stroke, have been hypothesised (Brown, Lutsep, Weinand, & Cramer, 2008; Brown & Pilitsis, 2006).

Two main strategies for using NIBS to modulate brain function can be distinguished: One aim is to increase cortical excitability or training-induced LTP-like mechanisms in the area of interest. Increasing the excitability of neurons in one brain region may promote improvements in performance possibly by facilitating LTP-like processes between activated neurons (Liebetanz et al., 2002). Practising certain behaviours, such as finger movements in the motor system, naturally heightens motor-cortical excitability (Garry, Kamen, & Nordstrom, 2004; Koeneke, Lutz, Herwig, & Ziemann, 2006). Therefore increasing excitability with brain stimulation, whether directly or indirectly, may provide a means of inducing a physiological state that supports acquiring novel skills (Floel & Cohen, 2009), or may even facilitate off-line learning (Reis et al., 2009). Additionally, facilitatory NIBS may then also indicate the functional significance of the stimulated area for the respective task.

Second, NIBS may be used to inhibit networks. Thus the behaviour under study will be disturbed in most set-ups, primarily providing evidence about the functional involvement of the specific area for the task under study. TMS can interfere with cognitive functions in two ways. A high-intensity TMS pulse may cause a synchronised high-frequency burst of discharge in a relatively large population of neurons that is terminated by a long-lasting GABAergic inhibition. The combination of artificial synchronisation of activity followed by depression effectively disrupts cognitive processes in the human brain, a phenomenon also described as a "virtual lesion". Smaller intensities of stimulation produce less activity; in such cases cognitive operations continue but are disrupted due to the added noisy input from the TMS pulse (Sandrini, Umilta, & Rusconi, 2011; Siebner, Hartwigsen, Kassuba, & Rothwell, 2009). A recent paper by Schwarzkopf and colleagues (Schwarzkopf, Silvanto, & Rees, 2011) used the stochastic resonance phenomenon to more closely examine how TMS affects neuronal processing. They were able to demonstrate that while online low-intensity TMS facilitates the detection of weak motion signals, higher TMS intensities lead to impaired detection. These findings support the notion that TMS acts by adding noise to neuronal processing. Importantly, the stochastic resonance effects may explain why TMS parameters that under certain conditions impair behaviour may also induce facilitation when the stimulated area is in a different, e.g., adapted or suppressed, state. Siebner and colleagues (2009) have described the phenomenon of "context dependency", implying that the response to a given TMS pulse or train depends on how excitable the cortex is at the time the stimulus is applied: If many neurons are close to firing threshold then more of them are recruited by the pulse than at rest. Additionally, note that even "truly inhibitory stimulation" can be used to improve brain function in certain settings, for example after unihemispheric stroke: Here, an area would be inhibited that interferes with performance, for example an "over-active" right hemispheric region in aphasic patients (see Medina et al., 2012). Down-regulation of this area would dampen inhibitory projections from this area to left-sided language relevant areas, releasing the injured language area from (over)inhibition of the other side, and thereby improving its function.

The combination of TMS with functional neuroimaging has expanded the potential of TMS for human brain mapping. Precise and reliable positioning of the TMS coil is achieved via frameless stereotaxic systems that base their navigation either on the participant's structural magnetic resonance imaging (MRI), functional MRI data, or use functional neuroimaging data from the literature, so-called "probabilistic approach". The latter assumes consistency across individuals in the location of task-related "activations" in standardised stereotaxic space. Recent studies by Sack et al. (2009), and Sparing et al. (Sparing, Buelte, Meister, Paus, & Fink, 2008) systematically evaluated the accuracy of four and five different localisation strategies, respectively. Both studies found the highest precision with fMRI-guided stimulation, which was accurate within the range of millimetres. For more details on methods and special characteristics of each localisation strategy, see (Sparing, Buelte, et al., 2008).

In this review we summarise the main studies on TMS and tDCS in the language domain in the non-aphasic brain. In the first part we describe proof-of-principle studies aimed at improving language processing, or learning within the language domain. In the second part we try to convey how these techniques in their inhibitory mode allow powerful insights about brain–behavioural relationships, but also causal interactions among brain regions (i.e., combination of NIBS with other neuroimaging techniques). We end by providing a conclusion section on both facilitatory and inhibitory approaches with regard to tDCS vs TMS, and presenting an outlook on future developments in this research area.

BRAIN STIMULATION INCREASING CORTICAL EXCITABILITY AND FUNCTION

Transcranial magnetic stimulation (TMS)

The first studies have been conducted with TMS. Mottaghy and colleagues used short trains of high-frequency rTMS with low stimulation intensity (20 Hz, intensity of 55% stimulator output, duration of 2 s, offline) (Mottaghy et al., 1999) in 15 young males to modulate object-naming latencies. rTMS trains were delivered to Wernicke's area, the right-hemisphere homologue of Wernicke's area, to Broca's area, or to the primary visual cortex. A total of 20 black-and-white line drawings, which the individuals had to name as quickly as possible, were shown immediately after the completion of rTMS and again 2 minutes later. Immediately after the end of a train over Wernicke's area, a significant shortening of naming latency was seen compared to naming without rTMS. No significant effects on picture naming were observed 2 minutes later or at any time after stimulation of the right-hemisphere homologues of Wernicke's area, Broca's area, or the visual cortex. Thus a brief facilitation of picture naming could be demonstrated for the first time with rTMS, but the effects were rather small, showed high inter-individual variability, and were only short lasting.

A number of subsequent studies have used facilitatory rTMS in healthy individuals to investigate the functional significance of brain areas, as suggested in imaging studies, to certain language tasks.

Andoh and colleagues (2006) showed that rTMS over Wernicke's area improved performance (decreased reaction times, RTs) on an auditory task of word recognition. Importantly, they used fMRI to first localise the areas of interest in individual participants: Sentences in native or foreign languages were presented to 12 healthy right-handed male volunteers during fMRI. Three-dimensional functional maps localised the posterior temporal activation (Wernicke) in each participant and MRI anatomical cortical landmarks were used to define Broca's pars opercularis (F3Op). A frameless stereotaxy system was used to guide the TMS coil position over Wernicke's and F3Op areas in each participant. Active and placebo randomised rTMS sessions were applied at 1 Hz (110% of motor threshold (MT), 10 min, online rTMS) during the same language-fragment-detection task. RT was significantly decreased by active rTMS compared to placebo over Wernicke's area, and was more decreased for native than for foreign languages. No significant RT change was observed for F3Op area. rTMS conditions did not impair participants' accuracy. The authors suggested that low-frequency rTMS over Wernicke's area can speed up the response specifically to a task tapping native language perception in healthy volunteers, a finding similar to what Mottaghy and colleagues had shown for high-frequency rTMS with rather low stimulation intensities.

To investigate the neural substrate of rTMS-induced improvements in word recognition task performance (as demonstrated for example in Andoh et al., 2006; Gough, Nobre, & Devlin, 2005), Andoh and Paus (2010) combined offline rTMS with fMRI acquired during the performance of a word recognition task. A total of 20 healthy right-handed males underwent fMRI scans before and after a session of 10-Hz rTMS (15 trains with an intertrain interval of 10 s; 100% of MT) applied outside the MR scanner. Functional MR images were acquired during the performance of a word recognition task that used English or foreign-language words. rTMS was applied over left posterior temporal area of Wernicke in one group of 10 participants, whereas the homologue region in the right hemisphere was stimulated in another group of 10 participants. Changes in task-related fMRI response (English minus foreign languages) and task performances (RT and accuracy) were measured in both groups and compared between pre-rTMS and post-rTMS. It was found that rTMS increased task-related fMRI response in the homologue areas contralateral to the stimulated sites. Behaviourally, rTMS decreased RT for the left TMS group only. These findings provide additional evidence about the compensatory role of the homologue areas in the contralateral hemisphere for preserving behaviour after neural interference.

Although the studies cited above provide evidence for the potential use of rTMS to facilitate language processing, long-term effects have not been investigated so far in the healthy brain; but see conclusion section for first small studies in aphasic patients.

Transcranial direct current stimulation (tDCS)

Several studies so far used tDCS to assess verbal working memory (WM). Fregni et al. (2005) first tested whether anodal tDCS modified performance in a sequential-letter WM task when administered to the dorsolateral prefrontal cortex (DLPFC). A total of 15 participants underwent a three-back WM task based on letters. This task was performed during sham and anodal stimulation (1 mA, 20 min) applied over the left DLPFC. Seven of these participants also performed the task with inverse polarity (cathodal stimulation of the left DLPFC) and anodal stimulation of the primary motor cortex (M1). The authors found that only anodal stimulation of left DLPFC, but not cathodal stimulation of left DLPFC or anodal stimulation of M1, increased the accuracy of the task performance when compared to sham stimulation of the same area. RTs were not changed by stimulation.

Ohn et al. (2008) more closely examined the time-dependent effect of tDCS on working memory (sequential-letter WM task), by studying the effects of both 20-min tDCS and 30-min tDCS. They applied anodal stimulation over the left PFC in a single-blind, sham-controlled, crossover study in 15 healthy participants. A three-back verbal WM task was performed before, during, and 30 minutes after 1 mA anodal or sham tDCS. Anodal tDCS, compared with sham stimulation, significantly improved WM performance. Accuracy of response was significantly increased after 20 minutes of tDCS application, and was further enhanced after 30 minutes of stimulation.

Another study examined modulation of WM performance specifically in patients with idiopathic Parkinson's disease (IPS), who are known to present with deficits in this domain (Boggio et al., 2006). A total of 18 patients (12 men and 6 women) performed a three-back WM task during active anodal tDCS of the left DLPFC, anodal tDCS of M1, or sham tDCS. In addition patients underwent two different types of stimulation with intensities of 1 and 2 mA, respectively. The authors found a significant improvement in WM, as indexed by task accuracy, after active anodal tDCS of the left DLPFC with 2 mA. The other conditions did not result in a significant task performance change.

A recent study (Zaehle, Sandmann, Thorne, Jäncke, & Herrmann, 2011) then looked more closely at the neural substrates underlying the effect of tDCS on WM performance. The authors used EEG to assess the effect of left prefrontal tDCS (1 mA, 15 min) on oscillatory brain activity in a verbal WM task, comparing anodal vs cathodal tDCS vs control. They found increased performance and increased oscillatory power in the theta and alpha bands with anodal and decreased performance as well as decreased oscillatory power in the theta and apha bands with cathodal tDCS, compared to control. It is worthwhile noting that in all studies on WM discussed so far, RTs were insensitive to tDCS.

tDCS was also used to modulate verbal fluency (Iyer et al., 2005). Here, Iyer and colleagues applied 20 minutes of anodal, cathodal, or sham tDCS to the left PFC in three groups of right-handed participants and looked at verbal fluency, as well as global measures of processing and psychomotor speed, and emotion. In one experiment ($n = 30$), the authors tested before and after 1 mA tDCS and monitored EEG in nine participants. In two other experiments using 1 mA ($n = 43$) and 2 mA ($n = 30$), the authors tested before and then starting 5 minutes after the onset of tDCS. They found that all participants tolerated the stimulation well. No significant effects on performance with 1 mA tDCS were noted. At 2 mA, verbal fluency improved significantly with anodal and decreased mildly with cathodal stimulation. There were no clinically significant effects on the other measures. Note that this group did not find EEG changes induced by tDCS in the specific experimental set-up.

tDCS has also been used to assess naming performance and verbal RTs. This is an ecologically important endeavour, because proper names are difficult to learn (McWeeny, Young, Hay, & Ellis, 1987); name recall is a function that elderly people complain about as being impaired, and it is prone to loss in memory decline (James, Fogler, & Tauber, 2008), possibly due to their sparse connectivity in the semantic network.

Sparing et al. tested whether 7 minutes of 2mA tDCS would enhance visual picture naming. A total of 15 healthy participants performed the task before, during, and after tDCS applied over the posterior perisylvian region (PPR), i.e., an area that includes Wernicke's area (Sparing,Dafokatis, & Meister, 2008). Four different sessions were carried out: anodal and cathodal stimulation of left PPR and, for control, anodal stimulation of the homologous region of the right hemisphere and sham stimulation. Participants responded significantly faster following anodal tDCS to the left PPR. No decreases in performance were detected. Likewise, Fertonani et al. explored the effects of tDCS on picture naming in young healthy participants (Fertonani, Rosini, Cotelli, Rossini, & Miniussi, 2010). Anodal, cathodal (2 mA each), and sham tDCS were applied to the left DLPFC before two picture-naming experiments, a preliminary study (expt 1, 8-min stimulation) and a main study (expt 2, 10-min stimulation). The results showed that anodal tDCS of the left DLPFC speeded up verbal reaction times after the end of the stimulation, whereas cathodal stimulation had no effect. The authors hypothesised that the cerebral network dedicated to lexical retrieval processing were facilitated by anodal tDCS to the left DLPFC, and that cortical plasticity mechanisms led to facilitation lasting beyond the end of the stimulation. Note that, in both studies, effects of tDCS were only found on RTs.

A study by Ross and colleagues (Ross, McCoy, Wolk, Coslett, & Olson, 2010) then tried to improve not only the RTs but also the accuracy of naming performance with tDCS. A total of 15 young adults received left anodal, right anodal (1.5 mA, 15 min), or sham stimulation of the anterior temporal lobes, while naming pictures of famous individuals and landmarks. Right anterior temporal lobe stimulation significantly improved naming for people but not landmarks.

Two recent studies examined the effects of tDCS on recognition memory in patients with Alzheimer's disease (AD) (Boggio et al., 2009; Ferrucci et al., 2008). First, Ferruci and colleagues examined 10 patients with probable AD, using recognition memory and visual attention tasks (Ferrucci et al., 2008). In a within-participant design, in three sessions, they delivered anodal, cathodal, or sham tDCS over the temporoparietal area. Tasks were tested at baseline and 30 minutes after tDCS ended. They found that after anodal tDCS, accuracy of the word recognition memory task increased, whereas it decreased after cathodal tDCS and remained unchanged after sham. Visual attention-reaction times also remained unchanged. Boggio and colleagues investigated the impact of anodal tDCS on recognition memory, WM, and selective attention in AD (Boggio et al., 2009). Ten patients received three sessions of anodal tDCS (left DLPFC, left temporal cortex, and sham stimulation) with an intensity of 2 mA for 30 minutes. At each session Stroop, Digit Span, and a Visual Recognition Memory (VRM) task were performed. They found a significant effect of stimulation condition on VRM, and post hoc analysis showed an improvement after temporal and prefrontal tDCS as compared with sham stimulation. There were no significant changes in attention as indexed by Stroop task performance.

Both studies concluded that tDCS may enhance a component of recognition memory, and suggested further studies with repeated tDCS in conjunction with other therapeutic interventions for treating patients with AD. However, patient numbers were small, effects only short lasting, and a very specialised task was used. Moreover, the most effective stimulation parameters are still unclear; in fact, 30 minutes of 2 mA tDCS might even lead to a saturation of the tDCS effects (Nitsche et al., personal communication).

In sum, a number of studies have now demonstrated improved naming functions in healthy individuals, as well as patients with MCI or AD, after anodal tDCS. Thus a possibly fruitful area for research emerges with regard to naming abilities in patients with post-stroke aphasia, in whom impaired word-retrieval (anomia) is the most frequent symptom, with little or now spontaneous improvement after the first 6 months (Bhogal, Teasell, & Speechley, 2003). Here tDCS could be an interesting adjuvant therapeutic device; see also outlook section.

In order to induce long-lasting changes in language performance, tDCS may have to be administered in conjunction not only with a performance measure (to then improve immediate performance), but rather concomitant to a learning task. The basic idea behind this combination is that tDCS would modulate the learning process as such, and the resulting learning effects could be retained over time.

This principle was first applied in the realm of language learning for acquisition of a novel vocabulary (Floel, Rosser, Michka, Knecht, & Breitenstein, 2008). Here stimulation was applied over the posterior part of the left perisylvian area (position CP5 of the International 10–20 EEG System) in 19 young right-handed individuals, while participants had to acquire a miniature lexicon of 30 novel object names. Every participant took part in one session of anodal tDCS, one session of cathodal tDCS (each 20 min of 1 mA), and one sham session in a randomised and double-blinded design with three parallel versions of the miniature lexicon. With anodal stimulation, participants showed faster and better associative learning as compared to sham stimulation. Mood ratings, RTs, and response styles were comparable between stimulation conditions. Importantly, transfer of the vocabulary into participants' native language was also significantly better after learning under anodal tDCS, compared to cathodal tDCS and sham.

A further study (de Vries et al., 2010) used tDCS to investigate the causal relationship between Broca's area and learning of a novel grammar. Here an artificial grammar task (so-called Reber grammar; Reber, 1967) was used, because it constitutes a well-established model for the acquisition of grammatical knowledge in a natural setting, and previous neuro-imaging studies had demonstrated that Broca's area is similarly activated by natural syntactic processing and artificial grammar learning. A total of 38 healthy participants participated in a between-participant design, with either anodal tDDS (20 min, 1 mA) or sham stimulation, over Broca's area during the acquisition of the grammar. In the subsequent classification task, detecting syntactic violations, and specifically those where no cues to superficial similarity were available, improved significantly after anodal tDCS, resulting in an overall better performance. A control experiment where 10 participants received anodal tDCS over an area unrelated to artificial grammar learning further supported the specificity of these effects to Broca's area. The results cannot be explained by better tDCS-induced WM performance during the acquisition phase, which was comparable between groups. This is the first study that demonstrated tDCS-enhanced facilitation of the acquisition of grammatical knowledge.

The findings on associative verbal learning were corroborated in 2010 by Fiori and colleagues (2010). The authors again investigated the potential of tDCS to enhance associative verbal learning in the healthy brain (additionally, they looked at three patients with stroke-induced aphasia; for more information see contribution by Holland & Crinion, 2012). tDCS (20 min, 1 mA) was applied over Wernicke's area (again position CP5 of the International 10–20 EEG System) while 10 healthy individuals learned 20 new "words" (legal nonwords arbitrarily assigned to 20 different pictures). Each list was associated with a different stimulation condition in a single daily session over three consecutive weeks with a 6-day inter-session interval. It was found that left anodal stimulation led to a significant facilitation in picture naming with regard to vocal response times and not to naming accuracy. The authors point out that their results show that tDCS improves performance not only during recognition of new words (Floel et al., 2008) but also during word retrieval.

The studies referenced above demonstrate the possibility of enhancing training effects within the language domain (vocabulary, grammar) by tDCS. These exciting possibilities are currently been exploited in small proof-of-principle trials in aphasic patients (see e. g., Baker, Rorden, & Fridriksson, 2010; Floel et al., 2011; for more details refer to Holland & Crinion, 2012).

BRAIN STIMULATION DIRECTLY INHIBITING EXCITABILITY AND FUNCTION

Transcranial magnetic stimulation

Again, TMS was the first NIBS technique used to inhibit linguistic functions in healthy individuals and in epileptic patients. Here several studies using high-intensity, high-frequency rTMS over left PFC demonstrated (mostly in small studies) that this type of stimulation induces short-term deficits in performance of linguistic tasks, even up to the so-called speech arrest.

In epileptic patients Pascual-Leone and colleagues used online rTMS of 25 Hz and train duration of 10 s to produce speech arrest (Pascual-Leone, Gates, & Dhuna, 1991). The coil was centred over 15 different positions on each side of the scalp in six patients, and rTMS trains were applied while the patients counted aloud. rTMS centred over left prefrontal areas induced reproducible speech arrest in all participants and counting errors in three when applied at lower intensities. There were no such speech disturbances by rTMS centred over the different positions on the right side. Intracarotid amobarbital test (IAT) demonstrated left hemispheric language dominance in all patients. However, subsequent studies, looking at much larger number of individuals (Claus et al., 1993; $n=44$), showed that online rTMS (trains of 50 Hz, 100% of stimulator output, duration of 500 ms) over the temporo-parietal cortex of healthy participants, although producing more errors on verbal comprehension than stimulation over the right hemisphere, showed large inter-individual variability, and did not induce speech arrest in all participants. Thus it was not able to reliably determine hemispheric language dominance with this technique.

The ultimate rationale for most of these early studies was to replace the invasive IAT for determining hemispheric language dominance in patients before undergoing surgery for intractable epileptic seizures. However, this aim has never been realised, probably due to the still high percentage of individuals who did not show clear-cut lateralised arrest of language functions by these procedures; or in whom it was not clear if the speech arrest actually stemmed from inhibition of linguistic processes, or rather from inhibition of the motor output of speech.

Flitman et al. then used a less-intensive stimulation paradigm to selectively modulate language processing, trying to avoid interfering with speech motor output. Online rTMS was performed during a picture-word verification task (target), and a frame verification task (control) (Flitman et al., 1998). Half of the trials were performed during rTMS (15 Hz, 120% of MT, duration of 3 s). The effects of rTMS on performance were evaluated at four scalp positions, left anterior, a mirror site on the right, and two positions in the left and right parietal region. Stimulation over the left deltoid muscle served as a control. Participants had less difficulty in making picture-word matching decisions during unstimulated compared with stimulated trials at the left anterior and posterior positions. No significant difference in accuracy was detected in the frame verification condition, but response times in the frame verification condition were longer with stimulation at the left anterior position. Thus rTMS of the dominant hemisphere seemed to affect linguistic processing independent of speech motor output. However, this set-up is certainly not sufficient for clinicians to determine the hemisphere of language dominance before epileptic surgery, and has not been used in this context.

A number of subsequent studies successfully used TMS to better understand the significance of functional activation in imaging studies, and their relationship to the effects that actual lesions (like stroke) of a certain area would have on the underlying function. Here a study by Knecht and colleagues looked at the effects of offline inhibitory rTMS on language function in individuals with right versus left versus bilateral pattern of language lateralisation, as shown on functional brain imaging. Low-frequency rTMS (1 Hz, 110% of MT, 10 min) was applied during a word generation task over left and right PFC in one group of healthy volunteers with left, one with right, and one with bilateral language lateralisation, as shown on functional imaging (Knecht et al., 2002). It was found that participants with a right-sided activation showed inhibited word generation by rTMS over right PFC, whereas participants with left-sided activation were inhibited by rTMS over left PFC. Participants with a bilateral pattern of language activation were not significantly affected by inhibition of either side. It was concluded that, in some people, language processing seems to be distributed evenly between the hemispheres. Thus unilateral disturbance can be compensated by the other hemisphere, possibly by an acute up-regulation of the non-stimulated hemisphere. No study has subsequently combined brain stimulation with functional imaging to further test this hypothesis in participants with bilateral activation on functional-imaging language tasks.

A number of other studies have likewise used off-line rTMS to study brain-behaviour relationships: Sparing and colleagues (2001) investigated whether low-frequency rTMS (1 Hz) or high-frequency rTMS (20 Hz) at subthreshold intensities is also capable of influencing picture naming. In 16 healthy right-handed male participants, trains of offline 1 Hz or offline 20 Hz rTMS were applied over Wernicke's area, Broca's area, or the primary visual cortex. The participants had to name 20 black-and-white line drawings, which were shown immediately after rTMS and again 2 minutes later. Naming latency could be facilitated only immediately after Wernicke's area stimulation at a frequency of 20 Hz and at an intensity of 55% of the maximal stimulator output, which was more than the motor threshold. All other stimulation procedures failed to influence naming latencies. These results indicate that language functions can be facilitated in healthy participants only by high-frequency rTMS with intensities at or above the motor threshold. Another study examined the differential effect of rTMS on articulation versus linguistic function: A number of studies have used online TMS to examine the causal relevance for, and interaction between, specific brain regions for aspects of language processing previously identified by brain-imaging techniques.

Nixon and colleagues (Nixon, Lazarova, Hodinott-Hill, Gough, & Passingham, 2004) used TMS to examine the role of the left inferior frontal gyrus (IFG) in phonological processing and verbal WM. They used two experiments in which rTMS was applied over the frontal operculum while participants performed a delayed phonological matching task, and compared disruption of this area either during the delay (memory) phase or at the response (decision) phase of the task. They found that rTMS delivered at a time when participants were required to remember the sound of a visually presented word impaired the accuracy with which they subsequently performed the task, while rTMS delivered later in the trial, as the participants compared the remembered word with a given pseudoword, did not impair accuracy. Their findings suggest that the opercular region of the IFG is necessary for the normal operation of phonologically based WM mechanisms.

Romero and colleagues (Romero, Walsh, & Papagno, 2006) used rTMS while participants performed two phonological judgements, thought to require only articulatory rehearsal without the contribution of short-term storage; a digit span, which involves both, short-term storage and articulatory rehearsal; and a pattern span as a control task, with rTMS over left BA 40, left BA 44, and the electrode location, and without rTMS. They found that RTs increased and accuracy decreased in the case of the phonological judgements and digit span after stimulation of both left sites, suggesting that BA 40, in addition to BA 44, is involved in phonological judgements.

Devlin and colleagues (Devlin, Matthews, & Rushworth, 2003) employed combined fMRI/TMS to investigate semantic functions in the left inferior prefrontal cortex (LIPC). First they demonstrated with fMRI that semantic and phonological processing activated a common set of areas within the LIPC. In addition there was a reliable increase in activation for semantic relative to phonological decisions in the anterior LIPC while the opposite comparison (phonological vs semantic decisions) revealed an area of enhanced activation within the posterior LIPC. A second experiment used TMS to temporarily interfere with neural information processing in the anterior portion of the LIPC to determine whether this region was essential for normal semantic performance. Both repetitive and single pulse TMS significantly slowed participants' reactions for the semantic but not for the perceptual control task, thus suggesting that anterior and posterior regions contribute to both semantic and phonological processing, albeit to different extents.

Pattamolik and colleagues (Pattamadilok, Knierim, Kawabata Duncan, & Devlin, 2010) investigated the neural mechanism that underlie the influence that learning to read and write has on the processing of spoken language. Participants performed an auditory lexical decision task in which the orthographic consistency of spoken words was manipulated and rTMS was used to interfere with either phonological or orthographic processing by stimulating left supramarginal gyrus (SMG) or left ventral occipitotemporal cortex (vOTC), respectively. The advantage for consistently spelled words was removed only when the stimulation was delivered to SMG and not to vOTC, providing strong evidence that this effect arises at a phonological, rather than an orthographic, level.

Yet another rTMS study (Papagno, Fogliata, Catricala, & Miniussi, 2009) explored the different neural correlates for processing concrete and abstract words. The effect of rTMS over left inferior frontal, bilaterally posterior-superior temporal, and left posterior-inferior parietal cortex were compared during a lexical decision paradigm. An interference on accuracy was found for abstract words when rTMS was applied over the left temporal site, while accuracy for concrete words decreased when rTMS was applied over the right temporal site. Accuracy for abstract words, but not for concrete words, decreased after frontal stimulation as compared to the sham condition, suggesting that abstract lexical entries are stored in the posterior part of the left temporal superior gyrus and possibly in the left IFG, while the regions involved in storing concrete items include the right temporal cortex.

Hartwigsen and colleagues used online dual-site TMS in a series of studies to examine the causal relevance of the SMG (Hartwigsen, Baumgaertner, et al., 2010) and the IFG (Hartwigsen, Price, et al., 2010) for modality-independent (i.e., auditory and visual) phonological decisions. TMS started 100 ms after word onset and consisted of four stimuli given at a rate of 10 Hz and intensity of 90% of active motor threshold. For SMG the authors found that the accuracy and RTs of phonological decisions were selectively disrupted relative to semantic and perceptual decisions when real TMS was applied over the left, right, or bilateral SMG. These effects were not observed for TMS over the angular gyri. Moreover they ascertained that the threshold intensity for inducing a disruptive effect on phonological decisions was identical for unilateral TMS over the right or left SMG. For IFG, they found that TMS of pIFG impaired RTs and accuracy of phonological but not semantic decisions for visually and auditorily presented words; these effects was not seen for TMS of aIFG. TMS over left, right, or bilateral pIFG disrupted phonological processing to a similar degree. Again, the intensity threshold for delaying phonological judgements was identical for unilateral TMS of left and right pIFG. In sum, they were able not only to demonstrate that right SMG and right pIFG contribute to accurate and efficient phonological decisions in the healthy brain, but also to demonstrate that neither left nor right SMG, or left and right pIFG, can compensate for one another if disrupted by NIBS.

Stewart and colleagues (Stewart, Walsh, Frith, & Rothwell, 2001) applied rTMS (10 Hz, 120% of MT, 10 s duration, online) to an anterior and a posterior prefrontal site of the right and left hemisphere each (posterior: area where speech disruption was associated with an EMG response from the mentalis muscle; anterior: about 5 cm anterior and 2 cm lateral to the previous site) while participants counted aloud and recited the days of the week, months of the year, and nursery rhymes. Analysis of EMG data and videotaped recordings showed that rTMS applied over a posterior site, lateral to the motor hand area of both the right and the left hemisphere, resulted in speech disruption that was accompanied by activation of the mentalis muscle, while rTMS applied over an anterior site on the left but not the right hemisphere resulted in speech disruption that was dissociated from activation of the mentalis muscle. This study specifically demonstrated that rTMS could actually inhibit language processing as such, and not merely the production of overt speech, as had been suggested after the earlier studies on speech arrest. Gough et al. (2005) used rTMS (10 Hz, 300 ms, 60% of stimulator output, online) to investigate the functional significance of differential activation in anterior and posterior left inferior frontal cortex (LIFC; identified on functional magnetic resonance imaging, fMRI) when the meaning and sound of words were being processed. They found that, relative to no stimulation, rTMS of the anterior LIFC selectively increased response latencies when participants focused on the meaning of simultaneously presented words but not when they focused on the sound pattern of the words. In contrast, the opposite dissociation was observed in the posterior LIFC, where stimulation selectively interfered with the phonological but not the semantic task. This double dissociation was regarded as further evidence for functionally distinct subdivisions of the LIFC, possibly due to separable cortico-cortical connections linking the anterior LIFC to temporal pole regions associated with semantic memory and the posterior LIFC to temporo-parietal regions involved in auditory speech processing.

A large number of studies have examined the effects of rTMS on encoding of verbal information, for review see (Floel & Cohen, 2007). Rossi and colleagues (2001) could demonstrate a dissociation between left and right prefrontal rTMS on encoding versus retrieval of verbal information, as had been suggested repeatedly by imaging studies and had led to the development of the hemispheric encoding/retrieval asymmetry "HERA" model (Tulving, Kapur, Craik, Moscovitch, & Houle, 1994). In the Rossi et al. study, rTMS (20 Hz, 90% of MT, 500 ms, online) in young individuals was used to transiently interfere with either left or right prefrontal brain activity during the encoding or retrieval of pictures showing complex scenes. It was found that DLPFC was crucial for the retrieval of the encoded pictorial information, whereas the left DLPFC was involved in encoding operations. Subsequently Rossi et al. (2004) extended their study to elderly individuals, in whom numerous neuroimaging findings had suggested that the lateralisation of PFC activation associated with episodic memory performance was reduced (hemispheric asymmetry reduction in older adults, "HAROLD" model; see Cabeza, 2002). Rossi and colleagues compared the effects of rTMS (20 Hz, 90% of MT, 500 ms, online) applied to the left or right DLPFC on visuospatial recognition memory in healthy participants below age 45, and above age 50. In young participants, rTMS of the right DLPFC interfered with retrieval more than left DLPFC stimulation. The asymmetry of the effect progressively vanished with ageing, as indicated by bilateral interference effects on recognition performance. Conversely, the predominance of left DLPFC effect during encoding was not abolished in elders. Their findings not only provide further support of greater bilaterally distributed encoding and retrieval in the ageing brain, but also suggest that the bilateral engagement of the DLPFC has a compensatory role, rather than being merely due to de-differentiation processes.

Focusing on encoding, Floel and colleagues (2004) probed the prefrontal asymmetry for verbal versus nonverbal material, which had been suggested by preceding imaging studies (Kirchhoff, Wagner, Maril, & Stern, 2000; Rugg, Otten, & Henson, 2002). The authors used rTMS (20 Hz, 90% of MT, 500 ms, online) to transiently interfere either with left or right PFC while participants memorised verbal and nonverbal items. It was found that encoding of verbal material was disrupted by left PFC stimulation, whereas encoding of nonverbal material was disrupted by right PFC stimulation. These results for the first time demonstrated a functionally relevant lateralisation of prefrontal contribution for verbal and nonverbal memory encoding.

In congenitally blind participants it was even possible to show that the left occipital pole is involved in verb generation, which is not the case in sighted controls (Amedi, Floel, Knecht, Zohary, & Cohen, 2004). In this study rTMS (20 Hz, 90% of MT, 500 ms, online) of left primary visual cortex (V1) reduced accuracy in a verb generation task, compared to control stimulation sites (PFC), as well as results seen in sighted controls. Further analysis revealed that the most common error produced by rTMS was semantic, while phonological errors and interference with motor execution or articulation were rare. Thus rTMS was able to provide functional evidence that the left V1 activation, seen in blind individuals during language tasks in imaging studies (Amedi, Raz, Pianka, Malach, & Zohary, 2003), actually indicates functional processing on this area. Thus further evidence was provided that V1, which is normally responsive to one sensory modality, can become sensitive to inputs from other sensory modalities, and even contribute to higher-cognitive language processing, in an activity-dependent manner if deprived from input from an early stage on.

As outlined in this section, a large body of studies have used inhibitory rTMS in the language domain to question causal brain–behaviour relationships, and to draw first conclusions about compensatory recruitment of additional brain areas if a specific area is disturbed.

Transcranial direct current stimulation

For tDCS, several studies using cathodal (inhibitory, given the results from neurophysiological studies) tDCS for assessing language functions have been negative, as reported alongside the positive study effects with anodal tDCS. In the study by Floel et al. (2008) cathodal tDCS (1 mA, 20min) over left Wernicke's area during acquisition of a novel vocabulary did not significantly affect learning in the young healthy volunteers, compared to sham (for more details on task see previous section). The study by Fregni and colleagues (2005) on tDCS in WM likewise looked at both anodal and cathodal effects on working memory performance (administered over left PFC). These authors also failed to observe a significant effect of cathodal tDCS (1 mA, 20 min). Moreover, Fertonani and colleagues (2010) did not find a significant effect of cathodal (2 mA, 10 min) tDCS over left DLPFC on verbal RTs in picture naming; Ross and colleagues (2010) could not show modulation of naming accuracy in naming pictures of famous individuals after cathodal tDCS (1.5 mA, 15 min) over right anterior temporal lobe. In the latter two studies, anodal tDCS over left DLPFC / right anterior temporal lobe had led to an increase in RTs or an increase in naming accuracy, respectively.

Other studies achieved a significant decrease in the language task under study with cathodal tDCS: Zaehle and colleagues (2011) could show both decreased performance on verbal WM, with a concomitant decrease in alpha and theta oscillatory power in EEG, using 1 mA, 15 min tDCS see section above for more details on this study. Vines and colleagues investigated the causal role of the left supramarginal gyrus in short-term pitch memory by comparing the effects of cathodal tDCS (1.2 mA, 20 min) when applied over the left or right supramarginal gyrus with sham, in 11 healthy individuals (Vines, Schnider, & Schlaug, 2006). Only cathodal tDCS over the left supramarginal gyrus decreased short-term pitch-memory performance. Ferruci and colleagues (2008) examined how the cerebellum is involved in the practice and proficiency of non-motor functions like language. The effects of tDCS over the cerebellum on the after-effects on the practice-dependent increase in the proficiency of a visual WM task were tested in 13 healthy young participants. In addition, the effects of cerebellar tDCS on visual evoked potentials (VEPs) were tested in four participants, and the effects of cerebellar tDCS on the visual WM task were compared to those elicited by tDCS delivered over the prefrontal cortex in five participants. The results showed that anodal or cathodal tDCS over the cerebellum impaired the practice-dependent improvement in the reaction times in the visual WM task. Because tDCS delivered over the prefrontal cortex induced an immediate change in visual WM, but left the practice-dependent proficiency unchanged, it was concluded that the effects of cerebellar tDCS were structure-specific. Since cerebellar tDCS left VEPs unaffected, its effect on visual WM therefore seems unlikely to arise from visual system involvement. Thus cathodal tDCS over the cerebellum seems to specifically impair the practice-dependent proficiency increase in visual WM. A study by Liuzzi et al. (2010) examined the involvement of the left motor cortex in learning of a novel action word lexicon, using cathodal tDCS. In combination with tDCS (1 mA, 20 min) over the left M1, participants learned a novel vocabulary of 76 concrete, body-related actions by means of an associative learning paradigm. Compared with a control condition with "sham" stimulation, cathodal tDCS reduced success rates in vocabulary acquisition, as shown by tests of novel action word translation into the native language. The analysis of learning behaviour revealed a specific effect of cathodal tDCS on the ability to associatively couple actions with novel words. In contrast, these effects were not found in control experiments, when tDCS was applied to the prefrontal cortex or when participants learned object-related words. These findings support the notion that left M1 is causally involved in the acquisition of novel action-related words. Elmer and colleagues (Elmer, Burkard, Renz, Meyer, & Jancke, 2009) examined the behavioural effects of right or left-hemisphere frontal tDCS while participants performed a short-term learning and subsequent long-term retrieval of auditory presented nouns. A total of 20 participants, divided into two groups, performed an episodic verbal memory task during anodal, cathodal (each 1.5 mA, 5 min), and sham current application on the right or left DLPFC. It was found that left-sided application of cathodal tDCS impaired short-term verbal learning when compared to the baseline. No tDCS effects were observed on long-term retrieval. These results provide further support that the left DLPFC is a crucial area involved in short-term verbal learning mechanisms, a result that has likewise been shown with facilitatory anodal tDCS. Moreover, the authors showed that tDCS delivery with an intensity of 1.5 mA to the DLPFC during short-term learning does not disrupt longer lasting consolidation processes that are mainly known to be related to mesial temporal lobe areas.

In sum, while a number of studies found inhibitory effects of cathodal tDCS, others did not. This dissociation of clear-cut cathodal effects on motor cortex excitability (Nitsche & Paulus, 2000) on the one hand, and non-consistent effects of cathodal tDCS on behavioural tasks on the other, has been noted for the motor domain as well, for example in a study on implicit motor learning that used both anodal and cathodal stimulation versus sham (Nitsche, Schauenburg, et al., 2003). Tentative explanations include the possibility that cathodal tDCS, not eliciting an action potential by itself (Nitsche & Paulus, 2000), is not strong enough to reliably suppress activity in a given area. Alternatively, compensatory activity in other brain regions may be responsible for the absence of behavioural effects. Systematic studies of behavioural effects of cathodal tDCS in combination with functional imaging techniques to elucidate compensatory activation in other brain regions need to be conducted to resolve this question.

CONCLUSIONS

In the healthy brain, NIBS has been used in its inhibitory form to delineate the functional significance of a particular brain region, and possibly its connections, for the respective language task under study. Another important area of NIBS research has been the use of proof-of principle studies to improve language processing and learning.

For the first, TMS, both in its single-pulse and its repetitive form, allows the modulation of a specific function within milliseconds (single-pulse) or the order of seconds (particularly high-frequency rTMS trains). Thus it is possible to influence individual items only in a continuous language paradigm. In this setting tDCS has the disadvantage of requiring longer stimulation times (usually in the order of at least 10–20 minutes; Nitsche & Paulus, 2001), and thus of only influencing a task in its entirety. Also, several studies have failed to demonstrate functional decline with cathodal tDCS in the language domain. Furthermore, the better focality of TMS, roughly described as 1 × 1cm with a figure-of-eight coil (Hallett, 2007), allows more specific targeting of a certain area. With tDCS the active electrodes of 5 × 5 cm or 5 × 7 cm, as used in the majority of studies so far, will lead to a larger stimulated brain area. Having said that, there is some focality with tDCS with regard to the centre of the stimulating electrode; see for example Wagner and colleagues for a head model of the induced current density with anodal tDCS (Wagner, Valero-Cabre, & Pascual-Leone, 2007). Also, smaller electrodes are becoming available for use: NeuroConn (Ilmenau, Germany) now offers electrodes in a number of sizes, ranging from square-shaped models of 10 × 10 cm to round-shaped models with a diameter of 2 cm. So far no results with regard to language processing have been published with these smaller electrodes, but such investigations, particularly if combined with concomitant fMRI recordings, will shed more light on improved focality of tDCS.

A different picture emerges for the second scenario, the use of NIBS for "therapeutic purposes"; that is, its use to enhance a certain function over an extended period of time. Note that, in healthy participants, these studies are only proof-of-principle but, with regard to language rehabilitation, of great potential interest. Here tDCS possesses several advantages: It is non-aversive, eliciting only a slight tingling under the electrodes. Next, it can be applied continuously and safely for up to 30 minutes (Gandiga, Hummel, & Cohen, 2006; Iyer et al., 2005; Nitsche et al., 2005), close to the typical duration of a session of rehabilitative treatment, and be administered in synchrony with training protocols (Baker et al., 2010; Floel et al., 2011). Moreover, for use in randomised, double-blind trials, real tDCS and sham tDCS elicit comparably minimal discomfort and duration of sensations in the absence of differences in attention or fatigue, and thus cannot be distinguished from sham by study participants or investigators (Gandiga et al., 2006; Iyer et al., 2005; Nitsche et al., 2005). Of course this advantage holds true not only for randomised trials in neurorehabilitation, but for cognitive neuroscience as well. The device is also easy to use, small (so can potentially be carried by a patient during a rehabilitation session), and relatively inexpensive. TMS, on the other hand, requires a unit to store and deliver a charge (called a capacitor), and an electromagnetic coil. A system can be cumbersome (resembling a small refrigerator), although some have shown that the entire system could be made portable and weigh less than 20 pounds (Huang et al., 2009). Applied above motor threshold it elicits rather unpleasant sensations on the scalp, and has been associated with seizure induction in the past (Hallett, 2007; Rossi, Hallett, Rossini, & Pascual-Leone, 2009). Even though safety guidelines have been developed and are continuously updated (Rossi et al., 2009), concerns still arise in vulnerable populations like stroke patients, limiting the method's potential use in this setting (Loo, McFarquhar, & Mitchell, 2008). Thus, even though there is some potential to more permanently modulate function with (r)TMS (Ziemann et al., 2008), as demonstrated in simple studies in motor and visual systems (Miniussi et al., 2008), as well as in first studies in neurorehabilitation (Martin et al., 2009; Naeser et al., 2005; Pape, Rosenow, & Lewis, 2006), its function on learning within the language domain still needs to be elucidated. The patient studies by Naeser and colleagues (Martin et al., 2009; Naeser et al., 2005), although demonstrating long-lasting effects (months) of repeated rTMS sessions on naming functions in chronic post-stroke aphasia, included only few patients and no sham control; see also Holland and Crinion (2012). Moreover, given the above outlined advantages of tDCS for the rehabilitative setting in general, it may be most fruitful to improve on tDCS parameters for this purpose.

One question that has been addressed in several studies, but is still handled differently in current studies, is whether the placement of the TMS coil, and/or the tDCS electrodes, requires individual brain-imaging studies to localise the area of interest. Several authors have held the placing of electrodes by the 10–20 international EEG system, particularly in tDCS studies that use large electrode sizes, to be sufficiently precise, and the use of EEG electrode has been shown to be an appropriate method of localisation by neuronavigation techniques (Herwig, Satrapi, & Schonfeldt-Lecuona, 2003). However, comparative studies with TMS (Sack et al., 2009; Sparing, Buelte, et al., 2008) found placement by concomitant fMRI-TMS approaches to provide the most precise results; for more details see section above.

A further interesting question that has only been touched upon so far in the motor system asks whether the genetic background of the individual with regard to common genetic polymorphisms determines the response to a specific NIBS protocol (Cheeran, Koch, Stagg, Baig, & Teo, 2010). Previous studies have demonstrated differential responses to both TMS and tDCS in carriers of the BDNF Val66Met polymorphism in the motor system (see, for example, Cheeran et al., 2008; Fritsch et al., 2010). Within the language domain these questions are currently being pursued in ongoing studies of our laboratory and others.

OUTLOOK SECTION

The future is promising for the use of NIBS techniques. First, for the advancement of understanding brain–behaviour relationships, new possibilities of combining TMS or tDCS with functional imaging techniques offer unique opportunities not only to address the functional significance of a brain area underlying the coil or electrode, but also to allow testing NIBS effects on an entire network. It will be possible to directly examine if and how other brain areas may compensate for an area that is inhibited. Here dual-site TMS may be employed; see for example studies by Hartwigsen and colleagues (Hartwigsen, Baumgaertner, et al., 2010; Hartwigsen, Price, et al., 2010). Moreover, if NIBS is used directly in the scanner, not only may behavioural compensation be assessed, but also functional activation in response to inhibition of a particular area. For tDCS, devices are now commercially available that can be used in the scanner environment (NeuroConn, Ilmenau, Germany).

Another exciting area pertains to the realm of neurorehabilitation. Here NIBS, particularly tDCS, may be used concomitantly to training protocols to enhance language reacquisition, a potential only touched upon in small patient studies so far. For more details on its use in aphasia, see Holland & Crinion (2012); for use in non-aphasic patients with specific deficits in language processing, like MCI, AD, or PD patients, see above.

REFERENCES

Amedi, A., Floel, A., Knecht, S., Zohary, E., & Cohen, L. G. (2004). Transcranial magnetic stimulation of the occipital pole interferes with verbal processing in blind subjects. *Nature Neuroscience*, *7*(11), 1266–1270.

Amedi, A., Raz, N., Pianka, P., Malach, R., & Zohary, E. (2003). Early 'visual' cortex activation correlates with superior verbal memory performance in the blind. *Nature Neuroscience*, *6*(7), 758–766.

Andoh, J., Artiges, E., Pallier, C., Riviere, D., Mangin, J. F., Cachia, A., et al. (2006). Modulation of language areas with functional MR image-guided magnetic stimulation. *Neuroimage*, *29*(2), 619–627.

Andoh, J., & Paus, T. Combining functional neuroimaging with off-line brain stimulation: Modulation of task-related activity in language areas. *Journal of Cognitive Neuroscience*, *23*(2), 349–361.

Baker, J. M., Rorden, C., & Fridriksson, J. (2010). Using transcranial direct-current stimulation to treat stroke patients with aphasia. *Stroke*, *41*(6), 1229–1236.

Bhogal, S. K., Teasell, R., & Speechley, M. (2003). Intensity of aphasia therapy, impact on recovery. *Stroke*, *34*(4), 987–993.

Boggio, P. S., Ferrucci, R., Rigonatti, S. P., Covre, P., Nitsche, M., Pascual-Leone, A., & Fregni, F. (2006). Effects of transcranial direct current stimulation on working memory in patients with Parkinson's disease. *Journal of the Neurological Sciences*, *249*(1), 31–38.

Boggio, P. S., Khoury, L. P., Martins, D. C., Martins, O. E., de Macedo, E. C., & Fregni, F. (2009). Temporal cortex direct current stimulation enhances performance on a visual recognition memory task in Alzheimer disease. *Journal of Neurology, Neurosurgery & Psychiatry*, *80*(4), 444–447.

Brown, J. A., Lutsep, H. L., Weinand, M., & Cramer, S. C. (2008). Motor cortex stimulation for the enhancement of recovery from stroke: A prospective, multicenter safety study. *Neurosurgery*, *62* (Suppl. 2), 853–862.

Brown, J. A., & Pilitsis, J. G. (2006). Motor cortex stimulation. *Pain Medicine*, *7*, S140–S145.

Cabeza, R. (2002). Hemispheric asymmetry reduction in older adults: The HAROLD model. *Psychology & Aging*, *17*(1), 85–100.

Cheeran, B., Koch, G., Stagg, C. J., Baig, F., & Teo, J. Transcranial magnetic stimulation: From neurophysiology to pharmacology, molecular biology and genomics. *Neuroscientist*, *16*(3), 210–221.

Cheeran, B., Talelli, P., Mori, F., Koch, G., Suppa, A., Edwards, M., et al. (2008). A common polymorphism in the brain derived neurotrophic factor gene (BDNF) modulates human cortical plasticity and the response to rTMS. *Journal of Physiology*, *586*, 5717–5725.

Chen, R., Classen, J., Gerloff, C., Celnik, P., Wassermann, E. M., Hallett, M., & Cohen, L. G. (1997). Depression of motor cortex excitability by low-frequency transcranial magnetic stimulation. *Neurology*, *48*(5), 1398–1403.

Claus, D., Weis, M., Treig, T., Lang, C., Eichhorn, K. F., & Sembach, O. (1993). Influence of repetitive magnetic stimuli on verbal comprehension. *Journal of Neurology*, *240*(3), 149–150.

de Vries, M. H., Barth, A., Maiworm, S., Knecht, S., Zwitserlood, P., & Floel, A. (2009). Electrical stimulation of Broca's area enhances implicit learning of an artificial grammar. *Journal of Cognitive Neuroscience*, *22*(11), 2427–2436.

Devlin, J. T., Matthews, P. M., & Rushworth, M. F. (2003). Semantic processing in the left inferior prefrontal cortex: A combined functional magnetic resonance imaging and transcranial magnetic stimulation study. *Journal of Cognitive Neuroscience*, *15*(1), 71–84.

Elmer, S., Burkard, M., Renz, B., Meyer, M., & Jancke, L. (2009). Direct current induced short-term modulation of the left dorsolateral prefrontal cortex while learning auditory presented nouns. *Behavioral & Brain Functions*, *5*, 29.

Ferrucci, R., Mameli, F., Guidi, I., Mrakic-Sposta, S.Vergari, M., Marceglia, S., et al. (2008). Transcranial direct current stimulation improves recognition memory in Alzheimer disease. *Neurology*, *71*(7), 493–498.

Fertonani, A., Rosini, S., Cotelli, M., Rossini, P. M., & Miniussi, C. (2010). Naming facilitation induced by transcranial direct current stimulation. *Behavioral Brain Research*, *208*(2), 311–318.

Fiori, V., Coccia, M., Marinelli, C. V., Vecchi, V., Bonifazi, S., Ceravolo, M. G., et al. (2010). Transcranial direct current stimulation improves word retrieval in healthy and nonfluent aphasic subjects. *Journal of Cognitive Neuroscience. Advance online publication.* doi:10.1162/jocn.2010.21579

Flitman, S. S., Grafman, J., Wassermann, E. M., Cooper, V., O'Grady, J., Pascual-Leone, A., & Hallett, M. (1998). Linguistic processing during repetitive transcranial magnetic stimulation. *Neurology*, *50*(1), 175–181.

Floel, A., & Cohen, L. G. (2009). Recovery of function in humans: Cortical stimulation and pharmacological treatments after stroke. *Neurobiology of Disease*, *37*(2), 243–251.

Floel, A., & Cohen, L. G. (2007). Contribution of noninvasive cortical stimulation to the study of memory functions. *Brain Research Reviews*, *53*(2), 250–259.

Floel, A., Meinzer, M., Kirstein, R., Nijhof, S., Deppe, M., Knecht, S., & Breitenstein, C. (2011). Short-term anomia training and electrical brain stimulation. *Stroke*, *42*, 2065–2067.

Floel, A., Poeppel, D., Buffalo, E. A., Braun, A., Wu, C. W., Seo, H. J., et al. (2004). Prefrontal cortex asymmetry for memory encoding of words and abstract shapes. *Cerebral Cortex*, *14*(4), 404–409.

Floel, A., Rosser, N., Michka, O., Knecht, S., & Breitenstein, C. (2008). Noninvasive brain stimulation improves language learning. *Journal of Cognitive Neuroscience*, *20*(8), 1415–1422.

Fregni, F., Boggio, P.S., Nitsche, M., Bermpohl, F., Antal, A., Feredoes, E., et al. (2005). Anodal transcranial direct current stimulation of prefrontal cortex enhances working memory. *Experimental Brain Research*, *166*(1), 23–30.

Fritsch, B., Reis, J., Martinowich, K., Schambra, H. M., Ji, Y., Cohen, L. G., & Lu, B. (2010). Direct current stimulation promotes BDNF-dependent synaptic plasticity: Potential implications for motor learning. *Neuron*, *66*(2), 198–204.

Gandiga, P. C., Hummel, F., & Cohen, L. G. (2006). Transcranial DC stimulation (tDCS): A tool for double-blind sham-controlled clinical studies in brain stimulation. *Clinical Neurophysiology*, *117*(4), 845–850.

Garry, M. I., Kamen, G., & Nordstrom, M. A. (2004). Hemispheric differences in the relationship between corticomotor excitability changes following a fine-motor task and motor learning. *Journal of Neurophysiology*, *91*(4), 1570–1578.

Gough, P. M., Nobre, A. C., & Devlin, J. T. (2005). Dissociating linguistic processes in the left inferior frontal cortex with transcranial magnetic stimulation. *Journal of Neuroscience*, *25*(35), 8010–8016.

Hallett, M. (2007). Transcranial magnetic stimulation: A primer. *Neuron*, *55*(2), 187–199.

Hartwigsen, G., Baumgaertner, A., Price, C. J., Koehnke, M., Ulmer, S., & Siebner, H. R. (2010). Phonological decisions require both the left and right supramarginal gyri. *The Proceedings of the National Academy of Sciences USA*, *107*(38), 16494–16499.

Hartwigsen, G., Price, C. J., Baumgaertner, A., Geiss, G., Koehnke, M., Ulmer, S., & Siebner, H. R. (2010). The right posterior inferior frontal gyrus contributes to phonological word decisions in the healthy brain: Evidence from dual-site TMS. *Neuropsychologia*, *48*(10), 3155–3163.

Herwig, U., Satrapi, P., & Schonfeldt-Lecuona, C. (2003). Using the international 10–20 EEG system for positioning of transcranial magnetic stimulation. *Brain Topography*, *16*(2), 95–99.

Holland, R., & Crinion, J. (2012). Can tDCS enhance treatment of aphasia after stroke? *Aphasiology*, *26*, 1169–1191.

Huang, Y. Z., Sommer, M., Thickbroom, G., Hamada, M., Pascual-Leonne, A., Paulus, W., et al. (2009). Consensus: New methodologies for brain stimulation. *Brain Stimulation*, *2*(1), 2–13.

Iyer, M. B., Mattu, U., Grafman, J., Lomarev, M., Sato, S., & Wassermann, E. M. (2005). Safety and cognitive effects of frontal DC brain polarization in healthy individuals. *Neurology*, *64*(5), 872–875.

James, L. E., Fogler, K. A., & Tauber, S. K. (2008). Recognition memory measures yield disproportionate effects of aging on learning face-name associations. *Psychology & Aging*, *23*(3), 657–664.

Kirchhoff, B. A., Wagner, A. D., Maril, A., & Stern, C. E. (2000). Prefrontal-temporal circuitry for episodic encoding and subsequent memory. *Journal of Neuroscience*, *20*(16), 6173–6180.

Knecht, S., Floel, A., Drager, B., Breitenstein, C., Sommer, J., Henningsen, H., et al. (2002). Degree of language lateralization determines susceptibility to unilateral brain lesions. *Nature Neuroscience*, *5*(7), 695–699.

Koeneke, S., Lutz, K., Herwig, U., Ziemann, U., & Jancke, L. (2006). Extensive training of elementary finger tapping movements changes the pattern of motor cortex excitability. *Experimental Brain Research*, *174*(2), 199–209.

Kuo, M. F., Paulus, W., & Nitsche, M. A. (2008). Boosting focally-induced brain plasticity by dopamine. *Cerebral Cortex*, *18*(3), 648–651.

Liebetanz, D., Nitsche, M. A., Tergau, F., & Paulus, W. (2002). Pharmacological approach to the mechanisms of transcranial DC-stimulation-induced after-effects of human motor cortex excitability. *Brain*, *125*(Pt 10), 2238–2247.

Liuzzi, G., Freundlieb, N., Ridder, V., Hoppe, J., Heise, K., Zimerman, M., et al. (2010). The involvement of the left motor cortex in learning of a novel action word lexicon. *Current Biology*, *20*(19), 1745–1751.

Loo, C. K., McFarquhar, T. F., & Mitchell, P. B. (2008). A review of the safety of repetitive transcranial magnetic stimulation as a clinical treatment for depression. *International Journal of Neuropsychopharmacoly*, *11*(1), 131–147.

Martin, P. I., Naeser, M. A., Ho, M., Doron, K. W., Kurland, J., Kaplan, J., et al. (2009). Overt naming fMRI pre- and post-TMS: Two nonfluent aphasia patients, with and without improved naming post-TMS. *Brain & Language*, *111*(1), 20–35.

McWeeny, K. H., Young, A. W., Hay, D. C., & Ellis, A. W. (1987). Putting names to faces. *British Journal of Psychology*, *45*, 215–226.

Medina, J., Norise, C., Faseyitan, O., Branch Coslett, H., Turkeltaub, P. E., & Hamilton, R. H. (2012). Finding the right words: Transcranial magnetic stimulation improves discourse productivity in nonfluent aphasia after stroke. *Aphasiology*, *26*, 1153–1168.

Miniussi, C., Cappa, S. F., Cohen, L.G., Floel, A., Fregni, F., Nitsche, M. A., et al. (2008). Efficacy of repetitive transcranial magnetic stimulation/transcranial direct current stimulation in cognitive neurorehabilitation. *Brain Stimulation*, *1*(4), 326–336.

Mottaghy, F. M., Hungs, M., Brugmann, M., Sparing, R., Boroojerdi, B., Foltys, H., et al. (1999). Facilitation of picture naming after repetitive transcranial magnetic stimulation. *Neurology*, *53*(8), 1806–1812.

Naeser, M. A., Martin, P. I., Nicholas, M., Baker, E. H., Seekins, H., Kobayashi, M., et al. (2005). Improved picture naming in chronic aphasia after TMS to part of right Broca's area: An open-protocol study. *Brain & Language*, *93*(1), 95–105.

Nitsche, M. A., Grundey, J., Liebetanz, D., Lang, N., Tergau, F., & Paulus, W. (2004). Catecholaminergic consolidation of motor cortical neuroplasticity in humans. *Cerebral Cortex*, *14*(11), 1240–1245.

Nitsche, M. A., Jaussi, W., Liebetanz, D., Lang, N., Tergau, F., & Paulus, W. (2004). Consolidation of human motor cortical neuroplasticity by d-cycloserine. *Neuropsychopharmacology*, *29*(8), 1573–1578.

Nitsche, M. A., Kuo, M. F., Karrasch, R., Wachter, B., Liebetanz, D., & Paulus, W. (2009). Serotonin affects transcranial direct current-induced neuroplasticity in humans. *Biological Psychiatry*, *66*(5), 503–508.

Nitsche, M. A., Liebetanz, D., Antal, A., Lang, N., Tergau, F., & Paulus, W. (2003). Modulation of cortical excitability by weak direct current stimulation: Technical, safety and functional aspects. *Supplements to Clinical Neurophysiology*, *56*, 255–276.

Nitsche, M. A., & Paulus, W. (2000). Excitability changes induced in the human motor cortex by weak transcranial direct current stimulation. *Journal of Physiology*, *527*(Pt. 3), 633–639.

Nitsche, M.A., & Paulus, W. (2001). Sustained excitability elevations induced by transcranial DC motor cortex stimulation in humans. *Neurology*, *57*(10), 1899–1901.

Nitsche, M. A., Schauenburg, A., Lang, N., Liebetanz, D., Exner, C., Paulus, W., & Tergau, F. (2003). Facilitation of implicit motor learning by weak transcranial direct current stimulation of the primary motor cortex in the human. *Journal of Cognitive Neuroscience*, *15*(4), 619–626.

Nitsche, M. A., Seeber, A., Frommann, K., Klein, C. C., Rochford, C., Nitsche, M. S., et al. (2005). Modulating parameters of excitability during and after transcranial direct current stimulation of the human motor cortex. *Journal of Physiology*, *568*(Pt. 1), 291–303.

Nixon, P., Lazarova, J., Hodinott-Hill, I., Gough, P., & Passingham, R. (2004). The inferior frontal gyrus and phonological processing: An investigation using rTMS. *Journal of Cognitive Neuroscience*, *16*(2), 289–300.

Ohn, S. H., Park, C. I., Yoo, W. K., Ko, M. H., Choi, K. P., Kim, G. M., et al. (2008). Time-dependent effect of transcranial direct current stimulation on the enhancement of working memory. *Neuroreport*, *19*(1), 43–47.

Papagno, C., Fogliata, A., Catricala, E., & Miniussi, C. (2009). The lexical processing of abstract and concrete nouns. *Brain Research*, *1263*, 78–86.

Pape, T. L., Rosenow, J., & Lewis, G. (2006). Transcranial magnetic stimulation: A possible treatment for TBI. *Journal of Head Trauma Rehabilitation*, *21*(5), 437–451.

Pascual-Leone, A., Gates, J. R., & Dhuna, A. (1991). Induction of speech arrest and counting errors with rapid-rate transcranial magnetic stimulation. *Neurology*, *41*(5), 697–702.

Pattamadilok, C., Knierim, I. N., Kawabata Duncan, K. J., & Devlin, J. T. (2010). How does learning to read affect speech perception? *Journal of Neuroscience*, *30*(25), 8435–8444.

Reber, A. S. (1967). Implicit learning of artificial grammars. *Journal of Verbal Learning & Verbal Behavior*, *5*, 855–863.

Reis, J., Schambra, H. M., Cohen, L. G., Buch, E. R., Fritsch, B., Zarahn, E., et al. (2009). Noninvasive cortical stimulation enhances motor skill acquisition over multiple days through an effect on consolidation. *The Proceedings of the National Academy of Sciences USA*, *106*(5), 1590–1595.

Romero, L., Walsh, V., & Papagno, C. (2006). The neural correlates of phonological short-term memory: A repetitive transcranial magnetic stimulation study. *Journal of Cognitive Neuroscience*, *18*(7), 1147–1155.

Ross, L. A., McCoy, D., Wolk, D. A., Coslett, H. B., & Olson, I. R. (2010). Improved proper name recall by electrical stimulation of the anterior temporal lobes. *Neuropsychologia*, *48*(12), 3671–3674.

Rossi, S., Cappa, S.F., Babiloni, C., Pasqualetti, P., Miniussi, C., Carducci, F., et al. (2001). Prefrontal cortex in long-term memory: An "interference" approach using magnetic stimulation. *Nature Neuroscience*, *4*(9), 948–952.

Rossi, S., Hallett, M., Rossini, P. M., & Pascual-Leone, A. (2009). Safety, ethical considerations, and application guidelines for the use of transcranial magnetic stimulation in clinical practice and research. *Clinical Neurophysiology*, *120*(12), 2008–2039.

Rossi, S., Miniussi, C., Pasqualetti, P., Babiloni, C., Rossini, P. M., & Cappa, S. F. (2004). Age-related functional changes of prefrontal cortex in long-term memory: A repetitive transcranial magnetic stimulation study. *Journal of Neuroscience*, *24*(36), 7939–7944.

Rossini, P. M., Barker, A. T., Berardelli, A., Caramia, M. D., Caruso, G., Cracco, R. Q., et al. (1994). Non-invasive electrical and magnetic stimulation of the brain, spinal cord and roots: Basic principles and procedures for routine clinical application. Report of an IFCN committee. *Electroencephalography & Clinical Neurophysiology*, *91*(2), 79–92.

Rugg, M. D., Otten, L. J., & Henson, R. N. (2002). The neural basis of episodic memory: Evidence from functional neuroimaging. Philosophical Transactions of the Royal Society London - Series B: *Biological Sciences*, *357*(1424), 1097–1110.

Sack, A. T., Cohen Kadosh, R., Schuhmann, T., Moerel, M., Walsh, V., & Goebel, R. (2009). Optimizing functional accuracy of TMS in cognitive studies: A comparison of methods. *Journal of Cognitive Neuroscience*, *21*(2), 207–221.

Sandrini, M., Umilta, C., & Rusconi, E. (2011). The use of transcranial magnetic stimulation in cognitive neuroscience: A new synthesis of methodological issues. *Neuroscience & Biobehavioral Reviews*, *35*(3), 516–536.

Schwarzkopf, D. S., Silvanto, J., & Rees, G. (2011). Stochastic resonance effects reveal the neural mechanisms of transcranial magnetic stimulation. *Journal of Neuroscience*, *31*(9), 3143–3147.

Siebner, H. R., Hartwigsen, G., Kassuba, T., & Rothwell, J. C. (2009). How does transcranial magnetic stimulation modify neuronal activity in the brain? Implications for studies of cognition. *Cortex*, *45*(9), 1035–1042.

Sparing, R., Buelte, D., Meister, I. G., Paus, T., & Fink, G. R. (2008). Transcranial magnetic stimulation and the challenge of coil placement: A comparison of conventional and stereotaxic neuronavigational strategies. *Human Brain Mapping*, *29*(1), 82–96.

Sparing, R., Dafotakis, M., Meister, I. G., Thirugnanasambandam, N., & Fink, G. R. (2008). Enhancing language performance with non-invasive brain stimulation: A transcranial direct current stimulation study in healthy humans. *Neuropsychologia*, *46*(1), 261–268.

Sparing, R., Mottaghy, F. M., Hungs, M., Brugmann, M., Foltys, H., Huber, W., & Topper, R. (2001). Repetitive transcranial magnetic stimulation effects on language function depend on the stimulation parameters. *Journal of Clinical Neurophysiology*, *18*(4), 326–330.

Stewart, L., Walsh, V., Frith, U., & Rothwell, J. C. (2001). TMS produces two dissociable types of speech disruption. *Neuroimage*, *13*(3), 472–478.

Strafella, A. P., Paus, T., Fraraccio, M., & Dagher, A. (2003). Striatal dopamine release induced by repetitive transcranial magnetic stimulation of the human motor cortex. *Brain*, *126*(Pt. 12), 2609–2615.

Tulving, E., Kapur, S., Craik, F. I. M., Moscovitch, M., & Houle, S. (1994). Hemispheric encoding/retrieval asymmetry in episodic memory: Positron emission tomography findings. *The Proceedings of the National Academy of Sciences USA*, *91*(6), 2016–2020.

Vines, B. W., Schnider, N. M., & Schlaug, G. (2006). Testing for causality with transcranial direct current stimulation: Pitch memory and the left supramarginal gyrus. *Neuroreport*, *17*(10), 1047–1050.

Wagner, T., Valero-Cabre, A., & Pascual-Leone, A. (2007). Noninvasive human brain stimulation. *Annual Review of Biomedical Engineering*, *9*, 527–565.

Zaehle, T., Sandmann, P., Thorne, J., Jäncke, L., & Herrmann, C. S. (2011). Transcranial direct current stimulation of the prefrontal cortex modulates working memory performance: Combined behavioural and electrophysiological evidence. *BMC Neuroscience*, *12*, 2.

Ziemann, U., Paulus, W., Nitsche, M. A., Pascual-Leone, A., Byblow, W. D., Berardelli, A., et al. (2008). Consensus: Motor cortex plasticity protocols. *Brain Stimulation*, *1*(3), 164–182.

APHASIOLOGY, 2012, 26 (9), 1103–1118

Using TMS to study the role of the articulatory motor system in speech perception

Riikka Möttönen[1] and Kate E. Watkins[1,2]

[1]Department of Experimental Psychology, University of Oxford, Oxford, UK
[2]Centre for Functional Magnetic Resonance Imaging of the Brain (FMRIB), University of Oxford, Oxford, UK

Background: The ability to communicate using speech is a remarkable skill, which requires precise coordination of articulatory movements and decoding of complex acoustic signals. According to the traditional view, speech production and perception rely on motor and auditory brain areas, respectively. However, there is growing evidence that auditory-motor circuits support both speech production and perception.
Aims: In this article we provide a review of how transcranial magnetic stimulation (TMS) has been used to investigate the excitability of the motor system during listening to speech and the contribution of the motor system to performance in various speech perception tasks. We also discuss how TMS can be used in combination with brain-imaging techniques to study interactions between motor and auditory systems during speech perception.
Main contribution: TMS has proven to be a powerful tool to investigate the role of the articulatory motor system in speech perception.
Conclusions: TMS studies have provided support for the view that the motor structures that control the movements of the articulators contribute not only to speech production but also to speech perception.

Keywords: Speech; Motor cortex; Motor evoked potential; Transcranial magnetic stimulation; Communication; Articulation.

The human auditory system plays a critical role in processing acoustic speech signals. Evidently it also supports speech production. Monitoring of one's own speech, i.e., the auditory consequences of one's own articulatory movements, is an essential aspect of speech production. For example, alterations of auditory feedback during speaking can affect motor control of articulatory movements (Houde & Jordan, 1998). Reactivity of the auditory regions in the superior temporal cortex is modified during articulation, presumably via efference copy mechanisms (Curio, Neuloh, Numminen, Jousmäki, & Hari, 2000; Numminen & Curio, 1999). Also, perception of acoustic speech signals is altered during execution of articulatory movements (Sams, Möttönen, & Sihvonen,

Address correspondence to: Dr Riikka Möttönen, Department of Experimental Psychology, University of Oxford, South Parks Road, Oxford, OX1 3UD, UK. E-mail: riikka.mottonen@psy.ox.ac.uk

KW is grateful to the late Laughlin Taylor for discussions of the data in patients with face area lesions, and to Ned Jenkinson for discussions of TMS effects. RM was supported by the Medical Research Council.

http://dx.doi.org/10.1080/02687038.2011.619515

2005). Thus it is uncontroversial that the auditory system interacts with the articulatory motor system during speech production. The idea that neural processing of acoustic speech signals produced by someone else would also rely on interacting auditory and motor systems is more controversial and the topic is under active debate among speech scientists (Hickok, 2010; Hickok, Houde, & Rong, 2011; Lotto, Hickok, & Holt, 2009; Pulvermuller & Fadiga, 2010; Rauschecker & Scott, 2009; Scott, McGettigan, & Eisner, 2009; Wilson, 2009).

A key question in speech perception research is how phonetic categories are extracted from acoustic speech signals. How is a listener able to perceive that a speaker said the word "cat" rather than, for example, "bat" or "cap"? And how is it possible that auditory tokens of "cat" produced by different speakers are perceived so similarly? Speech comprehension is a challenging task, because there is no one-to-one relationship between phonetic categories and acoustic features of speech sounds and the speech signals produced by different speakers in different contexts are highly variable. The speakers' articulatory gestures are somewhat less variable. For example, all speakers produce the word "cat" by first closing the vocal tract by moving the root of the tongue ("c"), then keeping the vocal tract open ("a") and finally closing it by moving the tip of the tongue ("t"). Generation of internal motor models of the speaker's articulatory movements could possibly facilitate speech comprehension, since there are physical constraints on how articulators can move during speech production. In other words, speech perception could (in addition to auditory processes) engage complementary motor processes that are involved in solving an inverse problem: Which articulatory movements could have produced a given acoustic speech signal?

The idea that the speech production system would be involved in speech perception is not new. A central claim in Liberman's motor theory of speech perception is that the listener detects the speaker's "neuromotor commands to the articulators" (or "intended articulatory gestures") from the acoustic signal (Galantucci, Fowler, & Turvey, 2006; Liberman, Cooper, Shankweiler, & Studdert-Kennedy, 1967; Liberman & Mattingly, 1985). The theory proposes that there is a one-to-one relationship between these neuromotor commands and the phonetic categories and, therefore, differing speech sounds can be mapped onto the same phonetic category. Thus, according to the motor theory, speech perception is inherently linked to speech production. However, most speech scientists have rejected this claim (and many other claims) of the motor theory; they consider speech perception to be a purely auditory process, not a motor or auditory-motor process (Diehl, Lotto, & Holt, 2004; Lotto et al., 2009). Moreover, neuroimaging studies of speech perception have consistently shown that speech processing specifically activates non-primary auditory regions in the superior temporal cortex, giving support for the view that the auditory system is critical for speech perception (e.g., Binder et al., 2000; Dehaene-Lambertz et al., 2005; Möttönen et al., 2006).

During the past decade, transcranial magnetic stimulation (TMS) has become a widely used method in cognitive neuroscience, because it can provide information that is complementary to neuroimaging. It has also provided speech scientists with new tools to investigate whether the motor system, not only the auditory system, could be involved in speech perception. Importantly, TMS has made it possible to test experimentally whether the neural circuits that control movements of the articulators are facilitated during listening to speech and whether these circuits contribute to speech perception. In this article we provide a review of studies that have used TMS to address these questions and discuss methodological and theoretical aspects of these studies. We also present new ideas of how TMS can be used in combination with other brain imaging techniques to investigate putative interaction between auditory and motor systems during speech perception.

USING TMS TO MEASURE MOTOR EXCITABILITY DURING SPEECH PERCEPTION

TMS activates cortical neuronal elements by electromagnetic induction. Single TMS pulses over the primary motor (M1) cortex elicit motor evoked potentials (MEPs) in the contralateral target muscles that can be measured using electromyography. The MEPs recorded from the hand muscles peak approximately 24 ms after the pulse, whereas MEPs recorded from the lip muscles typically peak approximately 10 ms after the pulse, because the pathway from the corticobulbar pathway to the lips is shorter that the corticospinal pathway to the hands. The TMS intensity that is required to elicit MEPs is highly variable across participants, most likely due to variability in the distance from the simulating coil to the cortical surface (Stokes et al., 2005). Moreover, within-participant variation in amplitudes of the MEPs is dependent on the functional state of the motor system. For example, TMS pulses of constant intensity elicit larger MEPs when the participant contracts the target muscle than when the muscle is relaxed. The MEP measurements provide an accurate tool to localise cortical representations of the different muscles in each participant and to normalise the TMS intensity across participants. Importantly, they also provide a direct measure (i.e., MEP amplitude) of the excitability of the motor pathways connecting muscles with their cortical representations.

Several studies have demonstrated that the amplitudes of MEPs recorded from the articulatory muscles increase during speech perception, suggesting that excitability of the motor representations of articulators is increased. Watkins, Strafella, and Paus (2003) stimulated the lip representation in the left M1 cortex and showed that these MEPs were enhanced while participants were listening to continuous speech or viewing a talking face (see also Sundara, Namasivayam, & Chen, 2001). In contrast, MEPs elicited by the stimulation of the hand representation in the left M1 or the lip representation in the right M1 were unchanged during auditory and visual speech perception, indicating that the increased motor excitability was specific to the lip representation in the left hemisphere. Moreover, excitability of the lip representation was not increased, while participants watched random movements of the upper face, eyes, and brows. Interestingly, when participants listened to environmental sounds, excitability of the lip representation was also increased in the left hemisphere (relative to right hemisphere) and there was no significant difference between this condition and speech conditions. This suggests that the increased motor excitability in the left articulatory motor system may not be specific to speech. Watkins et al. (2003) suggested that this increased excitability in the left M1 cortex was due to the fact that some environmental sounds could be imitated using the vocal tract (e.g., engine noise). In a similar way, listening to sounds that can be produced using hand actions (e.g., typing sounds) increases excitability in the hand area of the left M1 cortex (Aziz-Zadeh, Iacoboni, Zaidel, Wilson, & Mazziotta, 2010). Watkins et al. (2003) did not report statistical tests between a baseline condition (listening to white noise) and other experimental conditions. We have re-analysed the original data reported previously to provide the statistics for the comparisons of each condition with baseline. Lip MEPs induced by left M1 stimulation during both speech conditions were significantly increased from baseline; listening to speech: $t(7) = 2.18$, $p = .03$; viewing speech-related lip movements: $t(7) = 2.63$, $p = .02$, whereas non-speech conditions did not differ from baseline; listening to environmental noise: $t(7) = 1.46$; viewing eye movements: $t(7) = -0.19$. We have also analysed data from a group of 13 participants (the original eight published and an additional five new participants) and found the same pattern (see Figure 1); paired *t*-test with baseline condition: listening to speech: $t(12) = 2.33$, $p = .02$; viewing lip movements: $t(12) = 1.92$, $p = .04$; listening to environmental noise: $t(12) = 1.28$; viewing eye movements: $t(12) = -1.28$. It should be noted, however, that the difference between listening to speech and listening to environmental noise was not significant in this group either.

Recently, Murakami, Restle, and Ziemann (2011) showed that decreasing intelligibility of auditory speech (by adding noise) and visual speech (by speeding up the articulatory movements) further enhanced the facilitation of the MEPs recorded from the lips. This suggests that the engagement of the articulatory motor system is increased when speech signals are difficult to understand. This finding is in agreement with an idea that the motor system is a complementary system, which is recruited especially in challenging conditions (Wilson, 2009). It should be noted, however, that in this recent study (Murakami et al., 2011) and in the earlier study (Watkins et al., 2003) a significant facilitation was also found during listening to speech signals that were easy to understand, indicating that articulatory motor system is engaged even in optimal listening conditions (and without behavioural tasks). Murakami et al. (2011) also showed that listening to speech and viewing speech-related movements increased short-interval intracortical inhibition of lip MEPs using paired-pulse TMS. This may reflect inhibition of involuntary muscle activity during speech perception.

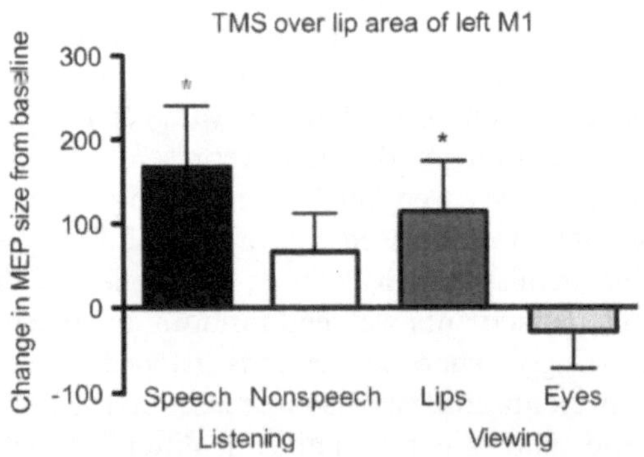

Figure 1. MEP sizes elicited in the contralateral orbicularis oris muscle by single-pulse TMS over the lip representation of left M1. Bars show the mean (+ standard error; *SEM*) change in MEP size (mV.ms) from a baseline condition (in which participants viewed visual noise and listened to white noise) while participants ($n = 13$) were listening to speech (Speech, mean = 167.65, *SEM* = 70.62) or environmental sounds (Nonspeech, mean = 67.10, *SEM* = 43.86), or viewing speech-related lip movements (Lips, mean = 114.33, *SEM* = 57.82) or eye and brow movements (Eyes, mean = –28.14, *SEM* = 41.86). MEP sizes (area under the curve of the rectified electromyographic recording) were adjusted for background contraction of the lip muscle using analysis of covariance (for details see Watkins et al., 2003). A paired *t*-test was used to compare MEP areas in each of these conditions with those in the baseline. The MEPs for the Speech and Lips conditions were significantly increased relative to the baseline condition (*$p < .05$).

Fadiga, Craighero, Buccino, and Rizzolatti (2002) examined whether the motor system is activated in an articulator-specific manner during speech perception. They stimulated the tongue representation in the left M1 while participants listened to Italian words that included phonemes that are articulated using the tongue (e.g., "r" in "birra") and words that are not articulated using the tongue (e.g., "biffa"). The tongue MEPs were found to be enhanced more during listening to words requiring tongue movements in production, compared to listening to other words. Moreover, the MEP enhancement was stronger for words than for pseudowords. Importantly, the pulses were delivered only 100 ms after the onset of the critical middle phoneme in this study, suggesting that the motor system is involved in speech processing at an early stage. Later, Roy, Craighero, Fabbri-Destro, and Fadiga (2008) replicated the earlier finding by showing that tongue MEPs elicited by pulses delivered 100 ms after the onset of the critical phoneme are sensitive to the articulatory features of the phonemes in pseudowords. The tongue MEPs elicited by pulses that were delivered later (200–300 ms after the onset) were sensitive to the frequency of the words (rare words caused stronger facilitation than frequent words), giving further support for the idea that lexical factors also affect the strength of motor excitability.

The increased size of MEPs elicited by stimulation of the cortical representation of the articulators reflects increased excitability in the motor pathways from the cortex to the brainstem nuclei innervating the lip and tongue muscles. Changes in excitability could therefore occur at either the cortical level in the upper motor neurons or at the level of the facial nucleus in the lower motor neurons. In addition, these changes in excitability could be brought about by inputs from other areas that are either cortical or subcortical. Paired-pulse TMS experiments over M1 representations have demonstrated muscle-specific modulation of intracortical facilitation and inhibition during observation of hand and arm movements (Strafella & Paus, 2000) and during auditory and visual perception of speech (Murakami et al., 2011). These findings support the view that the changes in excitability during action and speech perception occur at the cortical level rather than at the brainstem nuclei. The M1 cortex is not known to receive direct inputs from the visual or auditory cortex. It is thought that M1 cortical excitability is modulated instead by inputs from ventral premotor cortex (see Shimazu, Maier, Cerri, Kirkwood, & Lemon, 2004, for action observation in monkeys, and Cattaneo et al., 2005, for object perception prior to grasping in humans).Consistent with this suggestion, we found increased blood flow in ventral premotor cortex (Broca's area) correlated with motor excitability during speech perception in a combined positron emission tomography (PET) and TMS study (Watkins & Paus, 2004). Finally, the findings in speech perception studies that motor excitability is influenced by lexical factors (Fadiga et al., 2002, Roy et al., 2008) and is specific to the left hemisphere (Watkins et al., 2003) also point to a cortical origin for these effects, although additional subcortical influences cannot be ruled out.

Some functional MRI (fMRI) studies have also demonstrated that blood-oxygenation level dependent (BOLD) responses in the motor system are enhanced during listening to speech sounds (e.g., Callan, Callan, Gamez, Sato, & Kawato, 2010; Pulvermüller et al., 2006; Wilson, Saygin, Sereno, & Iacoboni, 2004). Increased BOLD responses in superior ventral premotor cortex are seen during listening to meaningless monosyllables, but this activity does not encompass primary motor cortex. Rather, it is localised to the border between primary motor (Brodmann area 4a) and premotor (Brodmann area 6) cortex (Wilson et al., 2004). Using region-of-interest (ROI) analyses, Pulvermüller and colleagues (2006) showed that listening to lip- or tongue-related phonemes modulated activity in the precentral gyrus in an articulator-specific manner. A dorsal ROI defined by activation to lip movement was more active during perception of lip-related phonemes ("p") than tongue-related phonemes ("t"), whereas a ventral ROI defined by activation to tongue movement showed the reverse pattern (Pulvermüller et al., 2006). Activity during speech perception in the primary motor cortex was not extensive and did not survive statistical thresholding in the whole-brain analysis. In a study comparing activations to an illusory percept "ta" created by the McGurk effect (combining auditory stimulus "pa" with visual stimulus "ka") with auditory or visual syllables "pa", "ta", and "ka", activation was found in the left precentral gyrus during listening to syllables (Skipper, van Wassenhove, Nusbaum, & Small, 2007). This activity was at the level of the lip representation and overlapped a region active in production of the same syllables.

It should be noted that many imaging studies using fMRI or PET, which have found enhanced activity in the temporal lobes during listening to speech, have failed to find such activity in the motor system. There are several possible explanations as to why imaging and MEP studies could have different sensitivities to speech processing in the motor system. First, there are likely to be individual differences in the somatotopic organisation and anatomy of the motor cortex (see Takai, Brown, & Liotti, 2010). Typically, in fMRI studies, brains of individual participants are registered into a standard space and the group-level statistical analyses are performed in this space. Therefore it is not surprising that the activations in the motor system do not reach statistical significance, if the individual representations of the articulatory organs (lip, tongue etc) do not overlap in the standard space (e.g., Pulvermüller et al., 2006). TMS studies avoid this problem by measuring MEPs from the same muscle in each participant (e.g., orbicularis oris for the lips) and separately localising the target regions in individuals. Second, the haemodynamic responses measured by PET and fMRI and motor excitability measured by TMS-induced MEPs may reflect different neural phenomena. This is supported by a recent fMRI study, which measured BOLD responses during anodal and cathodal transcranial direct current stimulation (tDCS) over the M1 cortex (Antal, Polania, Schmidt-Samoa, Dechent, & Paulus, 2011). Anodal tDCS increases and cathodal tDCS decreases motor excitability measured by TMS-induced MEPs from hand muscles (Nitsche & Paulus, 2000). However, neither anodal nor cathodal tDCS altered BOLD signals in the M1 cortex during rest (Antal et al., 2011). It should also be noted that in our combined TMS and PET study we did not find increased rCBF in the left M1 cortex during speech perception, even though simultaneously recorded lip MEPs were enhanced and there was no correlation between motor excitability and rCBF in the M1 cortex (Watkins & Paus, 2004). These studies demonstrate that haemodynamic responses are not necessarily increased when motor excitability is increased. Changes in motor excitability are thought to be caused by changes in the resting membrane potentials of motor neurons (Rothwell, 2008). These changes do not necessarily cause any changes in the level of spiking activity in the motor system. TMS-induced MEPs will, however, increase because a larger number of corticobulbar (or corticospinal) neurons are closer to the threshold and therefore fire (when the TMS pulse is delivered). The synchronisation of the TMS-induced motor neuron discharges or the number of repetitive discharges of individual neurons will also affect MEP size (Rösler & Magistris, 2008). Simply put, the changes in MEP size reflect changes in synaptic efficacy and membrane potentials of neuronal populations in the stimulated area due to excitatory or inhibitory inputs from other cortical areas (see above). The haemodynamic responses as measured by rCBF in PET or BOLD in fMRI reflect changes in energy consumption, but their underlying neuronal mechanisms are not fully understood. It is thought that they reflect both synaptic and spiking activity (see, e.g., Logothetis, 2002; Rosa, Kilner, & Penny, 2011). Possibly the neuronal mechanisms that increase the motor excitability do not consume enough energy in the M1 cortex to induce changes in haemodynamic responses.

In sum, recording of TMS-induced MEPs from articulatory muscles provides a powerful tool to study involvement of the motor system during speech perception. This method provides information that is complementary to fMRI and PET. To date, relatively few studies have used MEP measurements to study excitability of the articulatory motor regions during speech perception. This method has been more widely used to examine motor excitability changes in the hand area of the M1 cortex during action observation (e.g., Aziz-Zadeh et al., 2004; Fadiga, Fogassi, Pavesi, & Rizzolatti, 1995). In our opinion the full potential of this method has not been realised among speech scientists. For example, further studies using both speech and well-controlled non-speech signals are needed to clarify whether the excitability of the articulatory motor system is enhanced specifically during listening to speech or whether processing of some non-speech signals also engages this part of the motor system.

THE "VIRTUAL LESION" APPROACH: USING TMS TO DISRUPT SPEECH PERCEPTION

The single-pulse TMS studies demonstrate that the excitability of the articulatory motor system is increased during speech perception. They do not, however, indicate that the motor system contributes to speech perception. Therefore a number of recent studies have used TMS to induce temporary "virtual lesions" in the healthy human brain to address whether the motor system plays a causal role in speech perception.

Meister, Wilson, Deblieck, Wu, and Iacoboni (2007) applied low-frequency repetitive TMS (rTMS) over the premotor cortex in order to induce a temporary disruption (i.e., a "virtual lesion") in this area. After rTMS over the premotor cortex, participants were impaired at identifying syllables ("pa", "ta", and "ka") that were presented in noise. In contrast, participants were unimpaired in the control tasks (colour and tone discrimination) after rTMS over the premotor cortex. These findings were the first to provide confirmatory evidence that the motor system plays a causal role in speech perception.

We have also used low-frequency rTMS to induce temporary disruptions in the motor system to examine the role of the motor representations of articulators in the discrimination of speech sounds (Möttönen & Watkins, 2009). We stimulated the lip representations in the left M1 cortex for 15 minutes with rTMS and showed MEPs recorded from the lips were suppressed after rTMS, indicating reduced motor excitability. This rTMS-induced disruption impaired the ability of the participants to discriminate synthetic speech sounds that are lip-articulated from speech sounds that are not articulated by the lips ("ba" vs "da" and "pa" vs "ta", see Figure 2). However, this disruption did not influence their ability to discriminate two speech sounds that are not articulated by the lips ("ka" vs "ga" and "da" vs "ga", see Figure 2). An rTMS-induced disruption in the hand area of the M1 cortex did not impair discrimination of any speech sounds. These findings support the view that the motor representations of articulators contribute to discrimination of speech sounds in an articulatory-feature-specific manner. Possibly the disruption of the motor lip representation inhibited the generation of internal motor models that include lip movements. Discrimination

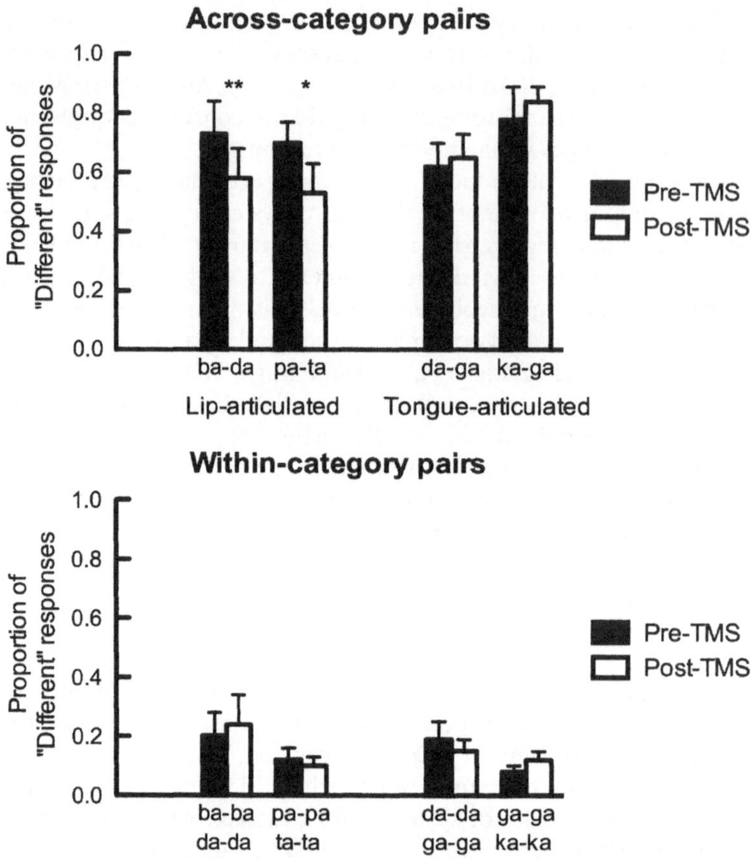

Figure 2. The effect of TMS-induced disruption in the motor lip representation on discrimination of speech sounds. Participants were presented with synthetic speech sounds from eight-step acoustic continua between two speech sounds. The pairs of sounds were categorised as "across-category" and "within-category" pairs based on the place of category boundaries that were determined for each participant individually. In the discrimination task participants were presented with pairs of synthetic speech sounds and asked to indicate whether the sounds are "same" or "different". Proportions of "different" responses are plotted. Participants gave more "different" responses when discriminating across-category pairs than within-category pairs, indicating categorical perception of speech sounds. Each participant performed the discrimination tasks before a low-frequency TMS train was applied over the lip representation in the left M1 cortex (pre-TMS) and after it (post-TMS). After TMS, participants were poorer in discriminating across-category pairs that included lip-articulated speech sounds ("ba" vs "da" and "pa" vs "ta") than before TMS. Discriminability of other pairs stayed stable. Data are from Möttönen and Watkins (2009). $^*p < .01$, $^{**}p < .001$.

of speech sounds that belong to the same phonetic category (i.e., within-category pairs) was poorer than discrimination of across-category pairs, although the acoustic distance between the sounds was the same (Figure 2). Enhanced discriminability of across-category pairs is a hallmark of categorical speech perception. The rTMS-induced disruption of the motor lip representation did not affect discrimination of any within-category pairs, which suggests that it relies completely on auditory mechanisms, not on motor or auditory-motor mechanisms.

Using a dual-pulse paradigm, D'Ausilio et al. (2009) have also found evidence supporting the contribution of the articulatory motor system to speech sound identification. Just before presentation of each syllable in noise the left motor cortex was primed by applying two TMS pulses either over the lip or tongue representation. The pulses over the lip area facilitated identification of the lip-articulated syllables ("pa"), whereas the pulses over the tongue area facilitated the identification of tongue-articulated syllables ("ta"). This TMS-induced facilitation was demonstrated by improved accuracy and reduced reaction times in this study. More recently, D'Ausilio, Bufalari, Salmas, Busan, and Fadiga (2011) have demonstrated that dual pulses over the representation of the larynx in the left motor cortex reduce reaction times in a demanding vocal pitch discrimination task (compared to dual pulses over the representations of the articulators), suggesting that this motor region, which controls phonation during speech production, may contribute to processing of pitch of speech sounds.

Sato, Tremblay, and Gracco (2009) found that low-frequency rTMS over the left ventral premotor cortex increased participants' reaction times in a phonetic segmentation task, but not in phoneme identification and syllable discrimination tasks. The accuracy was not affected by rTMS in any of the tasks. All speech stimuli were presented without noise in this study. These negative findings, and the fact that effects of TMS were weak and modulatory in previous studies (D'Ausilio et al., 2009; Meister et al., 2007; Möttönen & Watkins, 2009), have been interpreted in support of the argument that the motor system is not necessary for speech perception and that it contributes to speech perception only when listening conditions are compromised (Hickok et al., 2011; McGettigan, Agnew, & Scott, 2010). This may be true, but it is important to keep in mind the limitations of the TMS technique and the extent to which TMS can affect behaviour. TMS can add some noise to the neural processes in the stimulated areas but it cannot stop functioning of these areas. For example, during rTMS-induced disruption of the lip representation in the M1 cortex participants are able to move their lips and—unsurprisingly—comprehend clear speech (unpublished observations). Because the effects of TMS on neural processes in the stimulated areas are subtle, very sensitive behavioural tasks must be used to detect their behavioural consequences. Therefore in previous TMS studies noise has been added to the speech sounds (D'Ausilio et al., 2009; Meister et al., 2007) or their formant transitions have been manipulated (Möttönen & Watkins, 2009) to make their identification difficult. The fact that rTMS over the motor cortex can impair only slightly the ability to recognise and discriminate these types of speech sounds, but cannot abolish these abilities completely, should not be interpreted as indicating that the motor system plays a role only when speech perception is difficult.

Further TMS studies using variable tasks and speech stimuli (degraded and non-degraded) are needed to clarify in which conditions the articulatory motor system contributes to speech perception. In particular, it is not entirely clear whether in previous studies TMS-induced modulations in the motor system influenced task-related processes (such as phonemic segmentation and verbal working memory) that are not crucial for speech perception in everyday life. Furthermore, the tasks can force the participants to focus their attention on distinctive features of speech sounds. Therefore a challenge for further studies is to design tasks that are as natural as possible. Also, since previous TMS studies have focused on determining the role of the motor cortex in identification and discrimination of stop plosives that differ in the place of articulation, further studies focusing on other articulatory features of consonants (e.g., the manner of articulation) and vowels are needed.

Patients with real lesions have provided crucial information about the contributions of different brain areas to speech and language functions since the days of Wernicke and Broca. So far, studies in patients with lesions in the speech production system have reported somewhat conflicting evidence on these patients' speech perception abilities. Our attention was drawn to neuropsychological data obtained by Laughlin Taylor, who worked at the Montreal Neurological Institute and Hospital and tested patients before and after surgery in which part or all of their sensorimotor face area around the central sulcus was removed because of epilepsy (Taylor, 1979; see also Kolb & Wishaw, 2003, p. 417). Among other tests, Taylor presented patients with a phoneme identification task (Stitt & Huntington, 1969) requiring them to point to one of six letters corresponding to the six stop plosives ("p", "b", "t", "d", "k", "g") to indicate the phoneme heard. The phonemes were embedded in nonwords constructed by combining each with a nasal or a fricative sound and beginning and ending with the vowel "a" as in "f*a*ther" (e.g., "apma"," abma", "atma", "adma", "akma", "agma"). Taylor found that patients with lesions to the left face motor area recognised fewer than half of the stop plosives before (42%) and after (28%) the surgery. These patients performed worse than patients with lesions in the right face area (before: 63%, after: 68%), left frontal lobe patients (before: 58%, after: 58%) and left temporal lobe patients (before: 72%, after: 66%) even though the sizes of the surgical excisions in all of these groups were typically considerably bigger than the face area removals in the left hemisphere (Taylor, 1979; Kolb & Milner, 1981). Verbal fluency was also significantly impaired in patients with left central face area lesions compared even to left frontal lobe patients who also show restricted verbal fluency. However, they were unimpaired at performance of complex sequences of arm and facial movements (Kolb & Milner, 1981). This latter finding is somewhat at odds with a report that impairments in phoneme identification and in copying oral movements can be elicited by cortical stimulation of the same site, including stimulation of the left motor representation of the face (Ojemann & Mateer, 1979). Taylor concluded that the left face area patients "were unable to make effective use of phonetic elements of language" (Taylor, 1979, p. 171). It should be noted, however, that the central lesions extend to the post-central gyrus and although somatosensory function recovered well if the lesion was limited to the face area, we cannot rule out the effects on speech perception of damage to non-motor cortex. Also, the patients described by Taylor and Ojemann typically have had intractable epilepsy for many years and so may not be representative of normal brain organisation. These intriguing data warrant further investigations of similar patients with modern imaging techniques to determine exact lesion location and possible diaschisis.

There is also evidence that patients with Broca's aphasia are impaired in recognition of auditory words that are degraded, although their performance is at ceiling in recognition of non-degraded words (Moineau, Dronkers, & Bates, 2005). Patients with lesions encompassing the inferior frontal gyrus have also been suggested to be mildly impaired in syllable discrimination (Baker, Blumstein, & Goodglass, 1981; Blumstein, 2009; Blumstein, Baker, & Goodglass, 1977). On the other hand, speech perception can be relatively unimpaired in patients whose speech production abilities are severely impaired (for a review see Hickok, 2010; see also Bishop, Brown, & Robson, 1990, for speech perception in cerebral palsy). Recently a study in aphasic patients with fronto-parietal lesions (i.e., lesions in the "mirror neuron system") demonstrated that these patients show normal speech perception performance when non-degraded auditory stimuli are used (Rogalsky, Love, Driscoll, Anderson, & Hickok, 2011). These findings are consistent with the idea that the motor speech production system does not contribute to speech perception in optimal listening conditions.

The "virtual lesion" approach has several strengths relative to patient studies in the investigation of causal relationships between brain and behaviour (Walsh & Cowey, 2000). Damage to a particular region in patients is rare, and these natural lesions are often widespread and can lead to functional reorganisation of the brain over time. TMS-induced disruptions are temporary and more focal, which allows investigation of contributions of relatively small brain regions (e.g., motor representations of articulators) to behaviour in the healthy human brain. Due to these strengths, the "virtual lesion" approach has become a widely used tool. However, the approach has some limitations. First, it is not fully understood how TMS modulates neuronal processing (see, e.g., Classen & Stefan, 2008; Ziemann, 2010). Second, TMS can affect functioning of brain regions that are connected to the stimulated region. This complicates the conclusions that can be drawn from "virtual lesion" studies, because impairment in behaviour can be due to disrupted processing in connected brain regions, not only in the stimulated brain region (see, e.g., Siebner, Hartwigsen, Kassuba, & Rothwell, 2009). Moreover, it is difficult to estimate the size of the cortical area that is directly stimulated by a TMS coil. The (usually unwanted) spread of stimulation depends on the stimulation intensity. Therefore, it is advantageous to use as low intensity as possible in "virtual lesion" studies, which aim to test contributions of focal brain areas to behaviour (e.g., sub-threshold intensity when M1 is stimulated). Appropriate control sites and tasks are also essential. The articulatory-feature-specific effects found in our "virtual lesion" study suggest that it is possible to suppress excitability of motor representations in the M1 cortex selectively using sub-threshold low-frequency rTMS (Möttönen & Watkins, 2009). Also, rTMS over the hand motor representation have been shown to suppress specifically MEPs recorded from the hand, but not the biceps, muscles, suggesting that low-frequency rTMS can induce a relatively spatially focused effect within the cortex under the coil (Muellbacher, Ziemann, Boroojerdi, & Hallet, 2000).

COMBINING TMS WITH OTHER IMAGING MODALITIES: A NEW TOOL TO STUDY AUDITORY-MOTOR INTERACTIONS UNDERLYING SPEECH PERCEPTION

The combination of TMS with techniques that can measure brain activity in the whole brain makes it possible to look at how TMS affects neural processes outside the stimulated region (for reviews, see Driver, Blankenburg, Bestmann, Vanduffel, & Ruff, 2009; O'Shea, Taylor, & Rushworth, 2008; Ruff, Driver, & Bestmann, 2009). Since brain regions interact with each other during perceptual and cognitive processes, it is not surprising that "a virtual lesion" in one of the brain regions that are engaged in a process modulates functioning of other brains regions that are also engaged in the same process. Combining TMS with other techniques provides a new interesting method to examine how interacting brain regions support perception (e.g., Ruff et al., 2006, 2008).

There is strong evidence that the auditory regions in the superior temporal cortex play a critical role in speech perception. Therefore, in order to advance our understanding of the role of the motor system in speech perception, it is essential to investigate how the auditory and motor systems interact during speech processing and how this auditory-motor interaction supports speech perception. These questions can be addressed using a combination of TMS with brain imaging. For example, it is possible to examine influences of TMS-induced disruptions in the articulatory motor system on processing of speech signals in the superior temporal cortex using electroencephalography (EEG), magnetoencephalography (MEG), fMRI, and PET. Unpublished data from combined TMS and EEG experiments carried out in our laboratory demonstrate that TMS-induced virtual lesions in the articulatory motor cortex modulate automatic discrimination of speech sounds in the auditory system, suggesting the auditory and motor systems are functionally coupled during speech processing (Möttönen, Dutton, & Watkins, 2011). Importantly, the combination of TMS and neuroimaging also provides a tool to look at motor contributions to different stages of speech processing without demanding behavioural tasks that can be quite artificial and recruit additional processes that are not necessary for speech perception per se.

CONCLUSIONS AND FUTURE DIRECTIONS

The TMS studies reviewed here have provided consistent evidence that the articulatory motor system is activated during listening to speech and that it contributes to performance in various speech perception tasks. However, the role of the motor system in speech perception is not yet fully understood. Future experiments are needed to clarify in which conditions the motor system is recruited for processing of speech sounds. For example, the effects of the properties of speech signals, experimental tasks and selective attention need to be examined in future studies.

In this article we have focused mainly on studies that have looked at the role of the motor system in phonological processing of speech sounds. It is, however, likely that the motor system plays a role also in other aspects of speech and language processing, for example, in semantic processing of action-related words (Pulvermüller, 2005) and in turn-taking during conversations (Scott et al., 2009). One of the claims of Liberman's motor theory of speech perception was that "speech is special", meaning that only speech perception engages motor processes (Liberman et al., 1967; Liberman & Mattingly, 1985). It should be noted that according to current understanding this is not true, since the motor system seems to be involved in processing of variety of sensory inputs.

A few TMS studies have provided support for the idea that the speech sounds are processed in an articulatory-feature specific manner in the motor system. MEPs recorded from the tongue muscle are enhanced specifically during listening to words that include phonemes that are produced by closing the vocal tract with the tongue (e.g., "r"), but not during listening to words that that include phonemes that are produces by closing the vocal tract with the lips (e.g., "f") (Fadiga et al. 2002; Roy et al., 2008). Also, discrimination and identification of consonants that differ in place of articulation is affected in a somatotopic manner by stimulation of motor lip and tongue representations (D'Ausilio et al., 2009; Möttönen & Watkins, 2009). Although comparing consonants that differ in place of articulation has been a logical starting point and provided valuable information about motor influences on speech sound processing, categorising phonemes to lip- and tongue-articulated ones should be seen as a simplification. When continuous speech is produced, each articulator moves in time in a well-controlled manner and the articulatory movements are modulated by their phonetic context (due to coarticulation). Therefore it is a simplification to say, for example, that the lips would not be involved when dental and velar consonants (e.g., "t" and "k") are produced. In line with this the lip MEPs are enhanced even when TMS pulses are randomly delivered during continuous speech, not time-locked to "lip-articulated" phonemes (Murakami et al., 2011; Watkins et al., 2003). Further studies should try to take into account the complexity of the articulatory movements during speech production.

In face-to-face communication a speaker's articulatory movements are visible. Viewing these movements, not only listening to speech, activates the articulatory motor system (Campbell et al., 2001; Murakami et al., 2011; Watkins et al., 2003). It has been suggested that the motor system generates forward models of sensory consequences of observed articulatory movements (Kauramäki et al., 2010; Möttönen, Järveläinen, Sams, & Hari, 2005; Sams et al., 2005; Skipper et al., 2007; van Wassenhove, Grant, & Poeppel, 2005). It is likely that the motor system contributes to the integration of auditory and visual speech signals during audiovisual speech perception (Callan et al., 2003, 2004; Jääskeläinen, 2010; Ojanen et al., 2005). The articulatory motor system may have a stronger role in speech processing when the speaker's articulatory movements are visible compared to when the perceiver has to rely on auditory speech signals alone.

TMS has proven to be a powerful tool in investigating the role of the articulatory motor system in speech processing. This technique has potential to help speech scientists to address many remaining open questions in this research area. In our opinion, to better understand the role of the motor system in the processing of auditory and visual speech signals, it is important to investigate its interaction with the auditory system and other brain regions that support speech perception. Combining TMS with brain-imaging techniques offers a promising tool with which to examine these interregional interactions during speech processing.

REFERENCES

Antal, A., Polania, R., Schmidt-Samoa, C., Dechent, P., & Paulus, W. (2011). Transcranial direct current stimulation over the primary motor cortex during fMRI. *NeuroImage*, *55*(2), 590–596.

Aziz-Zadeh, L., Iacoboni, M., Zaidel, E., Wilson, S., & Mazziotta, J. (2004). Left hemisphere motor facilitation in response to manual action sounds. *European Journal of Neuroscience*, *19*(9), 2609–2612.

Baker, E., Blumstein, S. E., & Goodglass, H. (1981). Interaction between phonological and semantic factors in auditory comprehension. *Neuropsychologia*, *19*(1), 1–15.

Binder, J. R., Frost, J. A., Hammeke, T. A., Bellgowan, P. S., Springer, J. A., Kaufman, J. N., et al. (2000). Human temporal lobe activation by speech and nonspeech sounds. *Cerebral Cortex*, *10*, 512–528.

Bishop, D. V., Brown, B. B., & Robson, J. (1990). The relationship between phoneme discrimination, speech production, and language comprehension in cerebral-palsied individuals. *Journal of Speech and Hearing Research*, *33*(2), 210–219.

Blumstein, S. E. (2009). Auditory word recognition: Evidence from aphasia and functional neuroimaging. *Lang Linguistic Compass*, *3*(4) 824–838.

Blumstein, S. E., Baker, E., & Goodglass, E. (1977). Phonological factors in auditory comprehension in aphasia. *Neuropsychologia*, *15*, 19–30.

Callan, D., Callan, A., Gamez, M., Sato, M. A., & Kawato, M. (2010). Premotor cortex mediates perceptual performance. *NeuroImage*, *51*(2), 844–858.

Callan, D. E., Jones, J. A., Munhall, K., Kroos, C., Callan, A. M., & Vatikiotis-Bateson, E. (2004). Multisensory integration sites identified by perception of spatial wavelet filtered visual speech gesture information. *Journal of Cognitive Neuroscience*, *16*(5), 805–816.

Callan, D. E., Jones, J. A., Munhall, K. G., Callan, A. M., Kroos, C., & Vatikiotis-Bateson, E. (2003). Neural processes underlying perceptual enhancement by visual speech gestures. *Neuroreport*, *14*, 2213–2217.

Campbell, R., MacSweeney, M., Surguladze, S., Calvert, G., McGuire, P., Suckling, J., et al. (2001). Cortical substrates for the perception of face actions: An fMRI study of the specificity of activation for seen speech and for meaningless lower-face acts (gurning). *Brain Research Cognitive Brain Research*, *12*(2), 233–243.

Cattaneo, L., Voss, M., Brochier, T., Prabu, G., Wolpert, D. M., & Lemon, A. (2005). A cortoco-cortical mechanism mediating object-driven grasp in humans. *Proceedings of the National Academy of Sciences of the United States of America*, *102*(3), 898–903.

Classen, J., & Stefan, K. (2008). Changes in TMS measures induced by repetitive TMS. In E. M. Wassermann, C. M. Epstein, U. Zieman, V. Walsh, T. Paus, & S. H. Lisanby (Eds.), *The Oxford handbook of transcranial stimulation* (pp. 185–200). Oxford, UK: Oxford University Press.

Curio, G., Neuloh, G., Numminen, J., Jousmäki, V., & Hari, R. (2000). Speaking modifies voice-evoked activity in the human auditory cortex. *Human Brain Mapping*, *9*(4), 183–191.

D'Ausilio, A., Bufalari, I., Salmas, P., Busan, P., & Fadiga, L. (2011). Vocal pitch discrimination in the motor system. *Brain and Language*, *118*(1–2), 9–14.

D'Ausilio, A., Pulvermüller, F., Salmas, P., Bufalari, I., Begliomini, C., & Fadiga, L. (2009). The motor somatotopy of speech perception. *Current Biology*, *19*(5), 381–385.

Dehaene-Lambertz, G., Pallier, C., Serniclaes, W., Sprenger-Charolles, L., Jobert, A., & Dehaene, S. (2005). Neural correlates of switching from auditory to speech perception. *NeuroImage*, *24*, 21–33.

Diehl, R. L., Lotto, A. J., & Holt, L. L. (2004). Speech perception. *Annual Review of Psychology*, *55*, 149–179.

Driver, J., Blankenburg, F., Bestmann, S., Vanduffel, W., & Ruff, C. C. (2009). Concurrent brain-stimulation and neuroimaging for studies of cognition. *Trends in Cognitive Sciences*, *13*(7), 319–327.

Fadiga, L., Craighero, L., Buccino, G., & Rizzolatti, G. (2002). Speech listening specifically modulates the excitability of tongue muscles: A TMS study. *European Journal of Neuroscience*, *15*(2), 399–402.

Fadiga, L., Fogassi, L., Pavesi, G., & Rizzolatti, G. (1995). Motor facilitation during action observation: A magnetic stimulation study. *Journal of Neurophysiology*, *73*(6), 2608–2611.

Galantucci, B., Fowler, C. A., & Turvey, M. T. (2006). The motor theory of speech perception reviewed. *Psychonomic Bulletin Review*, *13*(3), 361–377.

Hickok, G. (2010). The role of mirror neurons in speech perception and action word semantics. *Language and Cognitive Processes*, *25*(6), 746–776.

Hickok, G., Houde, J., & Rong, F. (2011). Sensorimotor integration in speech processing: Computational basis and neural organisation. *Neuron*, *69*(3), 407–422.

Houde, J. F., & Jordan, M. I. (1998). Sensorimotor adaptation in speech production [see comments]. *Science*, *279*(5354), 1213–1216.

Jääskeläinen, I. P. (2010). The role of speech production system in audiovisual speech perception. *Open Neuroimaging Journal*, *4*, 30–36.

Kauramäki, J., Jääskeläinen, I. P., Hari, R., Möttönen, R., Rauschecker, J. P., & Sams, M. (2010). Lipreading and covert speech production similarly modulate human auditory-cortex responses to pure tones. *Journal of Neuroscience*, *30*(4), 1314–1321.

Kolb, B., & Milner, B. (1981). Performance of complex arm and facial movements after focal brain lesions. *Neuropsychologia*, *19*, 505–514.

Kolb, B., & Wishaw, I. Q. (2003). *Fundamentals of human neuropsychology* (5th ed.). New York, NY: Worth Publishers.

Liberman, A. M., Cooper, F. S., Shankweiler, D. P., & Studdert-Kennedy, M. (1967). Perception of the speech code. *Psychological Review*, *74*(6), 431–461.

Liberman, A. M., & Mattingly, I. G. (1985). The motor theory of speech perception revised. *Cognition*, *21*(1), 1–36.

Logothetis, N. K. (2002). The neural basis of the blood-oxygen-level-dependent functional magnetic resonance imaging signal. *Philosophical Transactions of the Royal Society of London B*, 357, 1003–1037.

Lotto, A. J., Hickok, G. S., & Holt, L. L. (2009). Reflections on mirror neurons and speech perception. *Trends in Cognitive Sciences*, *13*(3), 110–114.

McGettigan, C., Agnew, Z. K., & Scott, S. K. (2010). Are articulatory commands automatically and involuntarily activated during speech perception? *Proceedings of the National Academy of Sciences of the United States of America*, *107*(12), E42; author reply E43.

Meister, I. G., Wilson, S. M., Deblieck, C., Wu, A. D., & Iacoboni, M. (2007). The essential role of premotor cortex in speech perception. *Current Biology*, *17*(19), 1692–1696.

Moineau, S., Dronkers, N. F., & Bates, E. (2005). Exploring the processing continuum of single-word comprehension in aphasia. *Journal of Speech, Language and Hearing Research*, *48*(4), 884–896.

Möttönen, R., Calvert, G. A., Jääskeläinen, I. P., Matthews, P. M., Thesen, T., Tuomainen, J., et al. (2006). Perceiving identical sounds as speech or non-speech modulates activity in the left posterior superior temporal sulcus. *NeuroImage*, *30*, 563–569.

Möttönen, R., Dutton, R., Watkins, K. E. (2011). *Auditory-motor interaction supports automatic discrimination of speech sounds*. Manuscript in preparation.

Möttönen, R., Järveläinen, J., Sams, M., & Hari, R. (2005). Viewing speech modulates activity in the left SI mouth cortex. *NeuroImage*, *24*(3), 731–737.

Möttönen, R., & Watkins, K. E. (2009). Motor representations of articulators contribute to categorical perception of speech sounds. *Journal of Neuroscience*, *29*(31), 9819–9825.

Muellbacher, W., Ziemann, U., Boroojerdi, B., & Hallet, M. (2000). Effects of low-frequency transcranial magnetic stimulation on motor excitability and basic motor behaviour. *Clinical Neurophysiology*, *111*(6), 1002–1007.

Murakami, T., Restle, J., & Ziemann, U. (2011). Observation–execution matching and action inhibition in human primary motor cortex during viewing of speech-related lip movements or listening to speech. *Neuropsychologia*, *49*(7), 2045–2054.

Nitsche, M. A., & Paulus, W. (2000). Excitability changes induced in the human motor cortex by weak transcranial direct current stimulation. *Journal of Physiology*, *527*, 633–639.

Numminen, J., & Curio, G. (1999). Differential effects of overt, covert and replayed speech on vowel-evoked responses of the human auditory cortex. *Neuroscience Letters*, *272*(1), 29–32.

O'Shea, J., Taylor, P. C., & Rushworth, M. F. (2008). Imaging causal interactions during sensorimotor processing. *Cortex*, *44*(5), 598–608.

Ojanen, V., Möttönen, R., Pekkola, J., Jääskeläinen, I. P., Joensuu, R., Autti, T., et al. (2005). Processing of audiovisual speech in Broca's area. *NeuroImage*, *25*(2), 333–338.

Ojemann, G., & Mateer, C. (1979). Human language cortex: Localisation of memory, syntax, and sequential motor-phoneme identification systems. *Science*, *205*(4413), 1401–1403.

Pulvermüller, F. (2005). Brain mechanisms linking language and action. *Nature Reviews Neuroscience*, *6*(7), 576–582.

Pulvermüller, F., & Fadiga, L. (2010). Active perception: Sensorimotor circuits as a cortical basis for language. *Nature Reviews Neuroscience*, *11*(5), 351–360.

Pulvermüller, F., Huss, M., Kherif, F., Moscoso del Prado Martin, F., Hauk, O., & Shtyrov, Y. (2006). Motor cortex maps articulatory features of speech sounds. *Proceedings of the National Academy of Sciences of the United States of America*, *103*(20), 7865–7870.

Rauschecker, J. P., & Scott, S. K. (2009). Maps and streams in the auditory cortex: Nonhuman primates illuminate human speech processing. *Nature Reviews Neuroscience*, *12*(6), 718–724.

Rogalsky, C., Love, T., Driscoll, D., Anderson, S. W., & Hickok, G. (2011). Are mirror neurons the basis of speech perception? Evidence from five cases with damage to the purported human mirror system. *Neurocase*, *17*(2), 178–187.

Rosa, M. J., Kilner, J. M., & Penny, W. D. (2011). Bayesian comparison of neurovascular coupling models using EEG-fMRI. *PLoS Computational Biology*, *7*(6), e10002070.

Rösler, K. M., & Magistris, M. R. (2008). The size of motor-evoked potentials: Influencing parameters and quantification. In E. M. Wassermann, C. M. Epstein, U. Zieman, V. Walsh, T. Paus, & S. H. Lisanby (Eds.), *The Oxford handbook of transcranial stimulation* (pp. 77–90). Oxford, UK: Oxford University Press.

Rothwell, J. C. (2008). TMS measures and voluntary motor function. In E. M. Wassermann, C. M. Epstein, U. Zieman, V. Walsh, T. Paus, & S. H. Lisanby (Eds.), *The Oxford handbook of transcranial stimulation* (pp. 171–184). Oxford, UK: Oxford University Press.

Roy, A. C., Craighero, L., Fabbri-Destro, M., & Fadiga, L. (2008). Phonological and lexical motor facilitation during speech listening: A transcranial magnetic stimulation study. *Journal of Physiology, Paris*, *102*(1–3), 101–105.

Ruff, C. C., Bestmann, S., Blankenburg, F., Bjoertomt, O., Josephs, O., Weiskopf, N., et al. (2008). Distinct causal influences of parietal versus frontal areas on human visual cortex: Evidence from concurrent TMS-fMRI. *Cerebral Cortex*, *18*(4), 817–827.

Ruff, C. C., Blankenburg, F., Bjoertomt, O., Bestmann, S., Freeman, E., Haynes, J. D., et al. (2006). Concurrent TMS-fMRI and psychophysics reveal frontal influences on human retinotopic visual cortex. *Current Biology*, *16*(15), 1479–1488.

Ruff, C. C., Driver, J., & Bestmann, S. (2009). Combining TMS and fMRI: From 'virtual lesions' to functional-network accounts of cognition. *Cortex*, *45*(9), 1043–1049.

Sams, M., Möttönen, R., & Sihvonen, T. (2005). Seeing and hearing others and oneself talk. *Brain Research Cognitive Brain Research*, *23*(2–3), 429–435.

Sato, M., Tremblay, P., & Gracco, V. L. (2009). A mediating role of the premotor cortex in phoneme segmentation. *Brain & Language*, *111*(1), 1–7.

Scott, S. K., McGettigan, C., & Eisner, F. (2009). A little more conversation, a little less action – candidate roles for the motor cortex in speech perception. *Nature Reviews Neuroscience*, *10*(4), 295–302.

Shimazu, H., Maier, M. A., Cerri, G., Kirkwood, P. A., Lemon, R. N. (2004). Macaque ventral premotor cortex exerts powerful facilitation of motor cortex outputs to upper limb motoneurons. *Journal of Neuroscience*, *24*(5), 1200–1211.

Siebner, H. R., Hartwigsen, G., Kassuba, T., & Rothwell, J. C. (2009). How does transcranial magnetic stimulation modify neuronal activity in the brain? Implications for studies of cognition. *Cortex*, *45*(9), 1035–1042.

Skipper, J. I., van Wassenhove, V., Nusbaum, H. C., & Small, S. L. (2007). Hearing lips and seeing voices: How cortical areas supporting speech production mediate audiovisual speech perception. *Cerebral Cortex*, *17*(10), 2387–2399.

Stitt, C., & Huntington, D. (1969). Some relationships among articulation, auditory abilities, and certain other variables. *Journal of Speech and Hearning Research*, *12*, 576–593.

Stokes, M. G., Chambers, C. D., Gould, I. C., Henderson, T. R., Janko, N. E., Allen, N. B., et al. (2005). Simple metric for scaling motor threshold based on scalp-cortex distance: Application to studies using transcranial magnetic stimulation. *Journal of Neurophysiology*, *94*(6), 4520–4527.

Strafella, A. P., & Paus, T. (2000). Modulation of cortical excitability during action observation: A transcranial magnetic stimulation study. *Neuroreport*, *11*(10), 2289–1192.

Sundara, M., Namasivayam, A. K., & Chen, R. (2001). Observation-execution matching system for speech: A magnetic stimulation study. *Neuroreport*, *12*(7), 1341–1344.

Takai, O., Brown, S., & Liotti, M. (2010). Representation of the speech effectors in the human motor cortex: Somatotopy or overlap? *Brain and Language*, *113*(1), 39–44.

Taylor, L. B. (1979). Psychological asessment of neurosugical patients. In T. Rasmussen & R. Marino (Eds.), *Functional neurosurgery* (pp. 165–180). New York, NY: Raven Press.

van Wassenhove, V., Grant, K. W., & Poeppel, D. (2005). Visual speech speeds up the neural processing of auditory speech. *Proceedings of the National Academy of Sciences of the United States of America*, *102*(4), 1181–1186.

Walsh, V., & Cowey, A. (2000). Transcranial magnetic stimulation and cognitive neuroscience. *Nature Reviews Neuroscience*, *1*(1), 73–79.

Watkins, K., & Paus, T. (2004). Modulation of motor excitability during speech perception: The role of Broca's area. *Journal of Cognitive Neuroscience*, *16*(6), 978–987.

Watkins, K. E., Strafella, A. P., & Paus, T. (2003). Seeing and hearing speech excites the motor system involved in speech production. *Neuropsychologia*, *41*(8), 989–994.

Wilson, S. M. (2009). Speech perception when the motor system is compromised. *Trends in Cognitive Sciences*, *13*(8), 329–330; author reply 330–321.

Wilson, S. M., Saygin, A. P., Sereno, M. I., & Iacoboni, M. (2004). Listening to speech activates motor areas involved in speech production. *Nature Neuroscience*, *7*(7), 701–702.

Ziemann, U. (2010). TMS in cognitive neuroscience: Virtual lesion and beyond. *Cortex*, *46*(1), 124–127.

APHASIOLOGY, 2012, 26 (9), 1119–1130

Posterior middle temporal gyrus is involved in verbal and non-verbal semantic cognition: Evidence from rTMS

Paul Hoffman, Gorana Pobric, Mark Drakesmith, and Matthew A. Lambon Ralph

Neuroscience and Aphasia Research Unit (NARU), University of Manchester, Manchester, UK

Background: Left posterior middle temporal gyrus (pMTG) is reliably activated in functional neuroimaging studies of semantic processing and is frequently damaged in patients with comprehension impairments following stroke (e.g., Wernicke's aphasia). Its precise function remains elusive, however. Some researchers take the view that pMTG is a multimodal semantic area, involved in verbal and non-verbal semantic cognition. Others ascribe a lexical-semantic function to the region, positing that it is involved in mapping between phonology and conceptual knowledge.

Aims: We investigated whether pMTG was involved in non-verbal as well as verbal semantic cognition by using rTMS to induce temporary, focal "virtual lesions" to this region in healthy participants.

Methods & Procedures: Participants completed picture and word versions of a semantic association test before and after receiving 10 minutes of 1-Hz offline rTMS to left pMTG. They also completed a difficulty-matched visual decision task on scrambled pictures. An occipital lobe control site was stimulated in a separate session.

Outcomes & Results: TMS slowed responses to word and picture versions of the test to an equal degree. There was no slowing on a non-semantic visual-matching task, or following TMS to the control site.

Conclusions: These results indicate that pMTG is involved in both verbal and non-verbal semantic cognition. This region could be key to understanding the multimodal semantic deficits often observed following stroke.

Keywords: Conceptual knowledge; Semantic memory; Transcranial magnetic stimulation; Temporal lobe.

The left posterior middle temporal gyrus (pMTG) undoubtedly plays an important role in semantic cognition. It is one of the most reliably activated areas in functional imaging studies of semantic processing, as confirmed by its consistent appearance in meta-analyses of the neuroimaging literature on semantic cognition (Binder, Desai, Graves, & Conant, 2009; Cabeza & Nyberg, 2000; Indefrey & Levelt, 2004; Vigneau et al., 2006). It is also frequently damaged in patients with comprehension deficits

Address correspondence to: Dr Paul Hoffman, Neuroscience and Aphasia Research Unit (NARU), Zochonis Building, School of Psychological Sciences, University of Manchester, Oxford Road, Manchester, M13 9PL, UK. E-mail: paul.hoffman@manchester.ac.uk

The research was supported by an MRC programme grant (G0501632) and an NIHR senior investigator award to MALR.

http://dx.doi.org/10.1080/02687038.2011.608838

(Chertkow, Bub, Deaudon, & Whitehead, 1997; Hart & Gordon, 1990; Noonan, Jefferies, Corbett, & Lambon Ralph, 2010), with a large-scale lesion overlap analysis of 65 chronic patients identifying this region, rather than classical Wernicke's area (i.e., posterior superior temporal gyrus and sulcus), as critical for single-word comprehension (Dronkers, Wilkins, Van Valin, Redfern, & Jaeger, 2004). Despite the broad consensus on the importance of pMTG in semantic processing, a number of conflicting proposals have been put forward regarding its function. One school of thought holds that pMTG is important for mapping between the phonological forms of words and their meanings (Hickok & Poeppel, 2004, 2007; Indefrey & Levelt, 2004; Turken & Dronkers, 2011). On this view, pMTG acts as an interface between the auditory-phonological processing systems of Wernicke's area and semantic representations, which are thought to involve a number of distributed temporal lobe sites, including the anterior temporal lobes (Binder et al., 2009; Martin, 2007; Patterson, Nestor, & Rogers, 2007; Visser, Jefferies, & Lambon Ralph, 2010). This theory assigns pMTG a specific role in *lexical*-semantic processing, with no necessary involvement in non-verbal semantic cognition (e.g., object recognition, object use or comprehension of non-verbal sounds).

An alternative view is that pMTG is involved in semantic processing for both verbal and non-verbal stimuli. For example, many neuroimaging studies have reported that pMTG is strongly activated when retrieving knowledge of tools, leading to claims that pMTG is involved in the semantic representation of motion and actions (Devlin et al., 2002; Martin, 2007; Tranel, Martin, Damasio, Grabowski, & Hichwa, 2005). Importantly, pMTG activation is found for entirely non-verbal tasks, such as judgements about the functions and actions associated with pictured objects (Kellenbach, Brett, & Patterson, 2003) or matching pictures based on conceptual similarity (Kable, Lease-Spellmeyer, & Chatterjee, 2002). These findings suggest that pMTG is involved in aspects of the core conceptual representation of objects, rather than the linking between conceptual knowledge and the phonological representations of words.

A third possibility is that pMTG is involved in the executive control process that regulate access to conceptual knowledge (Jefferies & Lambon Ralph, 2006; Noonan et al., 2010; Whitney, Kirk, O'Sullivan, Lambon Ralph, & Jefferies, 2011). Although these control functions have been traditionally associated with inferior prefrontal regions (e.g., Badre & Wagner, 2007), neuroimaging studies have clearly demonstrated that activation in pMTG also varies with the control demands of semantic processing (Badre, Poldrack, Pare-Blagoev, Insler, & Wagner, 2005; Bedny, McGill, & Thompson-Schill, 2008; Gold et al., 2006; Noppeney, Phillips, & Price, 2004; Rodd, Davis, & Johnsrude, 2005; Whitney, Jefferies, & Kircher, 2011). For example, Thompson-Schill, D'Esposito, Aguirre, and Farah's (1997) seminal fMRI study of semantic selection demands revealed substantial activation in pMTG when participants selected among competing alternatives, in addition to the inferior prefrontal region that was the focus of the paper. More recently, Rodd et al. (2005) observed greater pMTG activation for comprehension of sentences containing ambiguous words (e.g., "the *shell* was *fired* towards the *tank*") relative to matched sentences with no such ambiguity. Ambiguous words are thought to require greater executive control because of the need to select the context-appropriate meaning of the word from all of its possible uses. It is unclear whether this control function is present for non-verbal as well as lexical stimuli, as very few imaging studies to date have manipulated control demands in a non-verbal semantic task.

In differentiating between these various functions, an important first step is to determine whether pMTG is implicated in non-verbal semantic cognition as well as lexical-semantic processing. On the surface, observations of pMTG activation for purely non-verbal semantic tasks appear to provide a conclusive answer to this question, but there are alternative interpretations. It has been noted by many researchers that activations in functional neuroimaging studies do not distinguish between regions that make a necessary contribution to the cognitive process of interest and those that are activated incidentally (e.g., Price & Friston, 2002). In this case one possibility is that when a picture of an object is processed its name is automatically retrieved, even if the judgement being made does not require any lexical processing. In this scenario pMTG activation could reflect the automatic name retrieval that occurs as a by-product of recognising the objects, rather than indicating a true role in multimodal semantic cognition.

Lesion studies do not suffer from this limitation: lesions to pMTG should only produce non-verbal semantic deficits if the function of this region is essential for non-verbal semantic processing. However, while there are a number of reports of non-verbal semantic deficits following pMTG damage, lesions to this area are usually accompanied by damage to bordering regions. Hart and Gordon (1990) identified three patients with pMTG damage who had multimodal semantic deficits, although their lesions also encompassed the adjacent superior temporal and inferior parietal cortex. Chertkow et al. (1997) found deficits on non-verbal semantic tasks in five of eight patients with verbal comprehension impairments. While the patients with multimodal deficits had damage to pMTG, which was not present in those with purely verbal impairments, posterior superior temporal and inferior parietal cortices were also affected. Finally, some patients with multimodal deficits in control and regulation of semantic knowledge (Corbett, Jefferies, Ehsan, & Lambon Ralph, 2009; Jefferies & Lambon Ralph, 2006; Noonan et al., 2010) have damage to pMTG, although this damage extends into inferior parietal cortex and the superior occipitotemporal region (BA37). Superior temporal cortex is heavily involved in verbal and non-verbal auditory processing (e.g., Leff et al., 2009; Saygin, Dick, Wilson, Dronkers, & Bates, 2003; Wise et al., 2001) and occipitotemporal cortex is implicated in high-level visual processing (e.g., Devlin, Jamison, Gonnerman, & Matthews, 2006; Kherif, Josse, & Price, 2011). As such, one possibility is that deficits on semantic tasks in these cases are due to perceptual impairments rather than genuine deficits in conceptual knowledge.

In the present study we used repetitive TMS (rTMS) to induce temporary "virtual lesions" in the left pMTG of healthy volunteers, and measured the effects on semantic association judgements for words and pictures. TMS produces focal stimulation that can be targeted at a precise area of cortex, avoiding the localisation problems in the neuropsychological literature. Moreover, a behavioural effect of TMS should only occur if the stimulated region is actively contributing to task performance. An additional benefit of rTMS is that performance in stimulated and non-stimulated conditions can be compared within the same healthy participants, which avoids effects of functional reorganisation that can occur in chronic brain injury (Walsh & Cowey, 2000). As in previous TMS studies of semantic processing (Gough, Nobre, & Devlin, 2005; Pobric, Jefferies, & Lambon Ralph, 2007, 2010a, 2010b) we measured both accuracy and reaction times but expected the relatively subtle effects of stimulation to be manifested as a slowing in reaction times, rather than an increase in error rates.

METHOD

Participants

A total of 14 staff and students from the University of Manchester took part (9 male; mean age = 21.1). All were right-handed, native English speakers. They had no history of neurological disease or mental illness and had normal or corrected-to-normal vision. All gave written informed consent and the experiment was reviewed and approved by the local ethics board. Participants were reimbursed for their participation.

Design

A 2 × 3 × 2 repeated-measures design was used, with site (left posterior middle temporal gyrus (pMTG) vs occipital pole), task (word semantic association vs picture semantic association vs pattern matching), and TMS (pre-TMS vs post-rTMS stimulation) as the three within-participants factors. We used the "virtual lesion" stimulation method in which a baseline level of behavioural performance is first obtained, then rTMS is delivered offline (with no concurrent behavioural task) and behavioural performance is probed immediately following stimulation during the temporary refractory period induced by the TMS. In pilot studies we have found that rTMS and the associated novel experience, irrespective of site of stimulation, can be highly alerting for participants and can produce a non-specific speeding in reaction times (Holland & Lambon Ralph, 2010). To control for any non-specific alerting effects we employed both a non-semantic control task (pattern matching) and a control stimulation site (occipital pole). In each session, each participant received stimulation to either pMTG or the control site, with the order counterbalanced across participants. Sessions were separated by an interval of at least 1 week.

Stimuli

Participants completed two semantic association tasks (words and pictures) and two visual control tasks (see Figure 1). The semantic tasks were created by combining trials from the Pyramids and Palm Trees test (PPT; Howard & Patterson, 1992) and the Camel and Cactus Test (Bozeat, Lambon Ralph, Patterson, Garrard, & Hodges, 2000). We supplemented these with 10 items from another semantic association task to give a total of 120 word and 120 picture stimuli. In order to maintain a two-choice format over the entire test, two of the three foils were discarded from each trial of the CCT. Stimuli for the visual matching control task were created by scrambling the picture and word images using the Java Runtime Environment (www.SunMicrosystems.com). Pictures were divided into 80 pieces and words into 15 pieces and these were re-assembled at random.

Procedure

A PC running with a 15-inch monitor and E-Prime software (Psychology Software Tools Inc., Pittsburgh, USA) controlled the presentation of stimuli and recording of the responses. Participants completed two sessions and performed all four experimental tasks twice in each session. Each session began with a series of practice trials for all

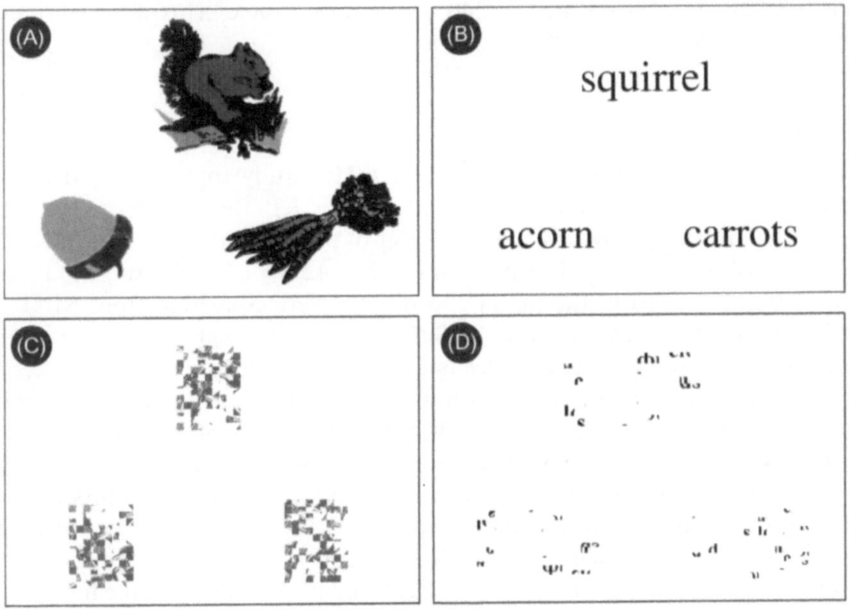

Figure 1. Experimental tasks. (A) and (B) show picture and word semantic association tasks and (C) and (D) show the corresponding mirror-image matching tasks. To view this figure in colour, please see the online issue of the journal.

four tasks, followed by pre-TMS task performance, 10 minutes of rTMS (see below), and post-TMS task performance.

In a single session participants saw all 120 trials from the combined PPT/CCT set, half as pictures and the remaining half as words. This order was counterbalanced across stimulation sites. There was no repetition of stimuli within a session but, across sessions, each trial was seen once in verbal and once in pictorial form. Experimental trials were presented in a random order in four blocks of 30 trials (pictures, words, scrambled pictures, and scrambled words). All blocks were randomised across participants. A fixation point appeared on the screen for 500 ms to signal the start of each trial. Stimuli were presented until response or for a maximum of 3000 ms followed by a blank screen interval of 500 ms. In semantic association trials participants were shown a probe picture/word and two choice and indicated which of the two choice stimuli was more closely related to the probe (see Figure 1). In the pattern-matching task participants were presented with three scrambled images and they had to indicate which of the two choice patterns was a mirror image of the probe. Pilot testing indicated that this demanding visual task yielded reaction times comparable to the semantic tasks. Participants indicated responses by pressing with the right hand one of two designated keys on a keyboard.

Anatomical MRI acquisition

Stimulation sites were selected using 3D anatomical images acquired using a 3T Philips MR Achieva scanner (Philips Electronics, The Netherlands). MRI scanning parameters included a slice thickness of 0.9 mm, a field of view of 24 cm, and an acquisition matrix of 256 × 256 × 240. A conjugate synthesis in combination with an interleaved acquisition resulted in 240 contiguous double-echo slices whose voxel dimensions were 0.94 × 0.94 × 0.9mm.

Selection of TMS site

The stimulation site was taken from a recent fMRI study that employed the same semantic and control tasks as the present study (Visser, Jefferies, Embleton, & Lambon Ralph, 2011). This study revealed a large cluster of pMTG activation for the semantic over control task contrast, with a peak at [−57, −42, −3] (see Figure 2). To locate this site in each participant, the target coordinates were converted from MNI space into each participant's native space using SPM5. Their T1-weighted scan was then co-registered with their scalp using an Ascension minibird magnetic tracking system and MRIreg software (http://www.cabiatl.com/mricro/mricro/mrireg/index.html) and the appropriate site marked on the scalp. Eight fiducial markers present during the scan (oil capsules attached to nasion, vertex, inion, tip of the nose, left/right mastoids, and left/right tragus during scanning) were used during the co-registration process.

A middle occipital stimulation site (occipital pole) was also employed as a site to control for possible non-specific visual effects and also for general arousal effects of TMS induced by somatosensory and acoustic artefacts. According to the international 10–20 electrode system, this site corresponds to the POz location.

Stimulation parameters

A MagStim Rapid2 (Magstim Co., Whitland, UK) stimulator with two external boosters was used (maximum output approx. 2.2 Tesla). Magnetic stimulation was applied using a 70-mm figure-of-eight coil. Individual motor threshold (MT) was determined for every participant prior to each session. Motor threshold was defined as a minimal intensity of stimulation capable of inducing contraction of the contralateral abductor

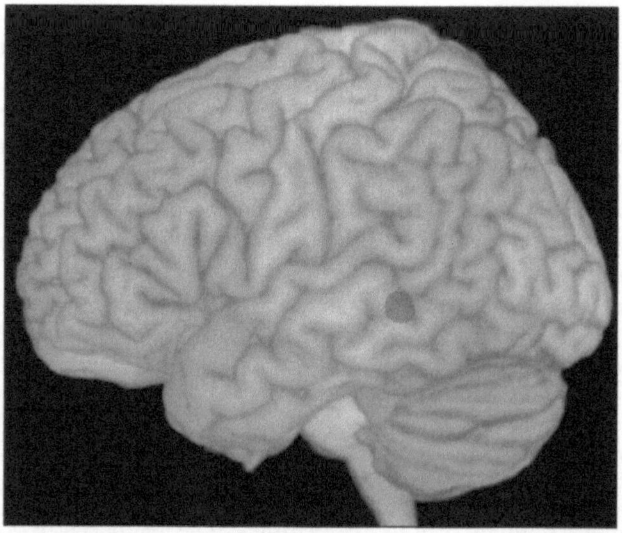

Figure 2. pMTG stimulation site [−57 −42 −3]. To view this figure in colour, please see the online issue of the journal.

pollicis brevis muscle at the optimal scalp position. The average MT was 55% of the maximal stimulator output and the average stimulation intensity during rTMS was 63%. Repetitive pulse TMS (rTMS) was delivered off-line for 10 min at 1 Hz (600 s at 120% motor threshold level) applied to either pMTG or occipital pole. This TMS protocol has been shown to produce behavioural effects that last at least 5 minutes following stimulation (Hilgetag, Theoret, & Pascual-Leone, 2001; Kosslyn et al., 1999). Pilot testing indicated that most participants completed the experimental task within 5 minutes.

RESULTS

Reaction times

There were six stimuli for which fewer than 50% of participants responded correctly. These trials were excluded from all analyses. To analyse reaction times, outliers more two standard deviations longer than a participant's mean in any condition were excluded (5% of trials). There was no significant difference between scrambled pictures and scrambled words ($p > .05$) so these were collapsed into a single control condition. Reaction times are shown in Figure 3. They were subjected to a $3 \times 2 \times 2$ repeated-measures ANOVA that included task, site, and TMS as within-participants factors. There were no main effects but there was a significant task × TMS interaction, $F(2, 26) = 14.4$, $p < .001$, and the site × TMS interaction approached significance, $F(1, 13) = 3.79$, $p = .073$. The task × TMS interaction occurred because participants reliably sped up on the control task following TMS, whereas no such effect was seen on semantic tasks. Performance on the control task was faster following stimulation of pMTG, $t(13) = 3.21$, $p < .01$, and occipital pole, $t(13) = 3.64$, $p < .01$. As this speeding effect was seen for both sites, it probably reflects a practice effect as a result of performing the task twice in a single session, rather than a specific effect of rTMS. There was no speeding for the semantic tasks. Instead, RTs to picture and word stimuli were

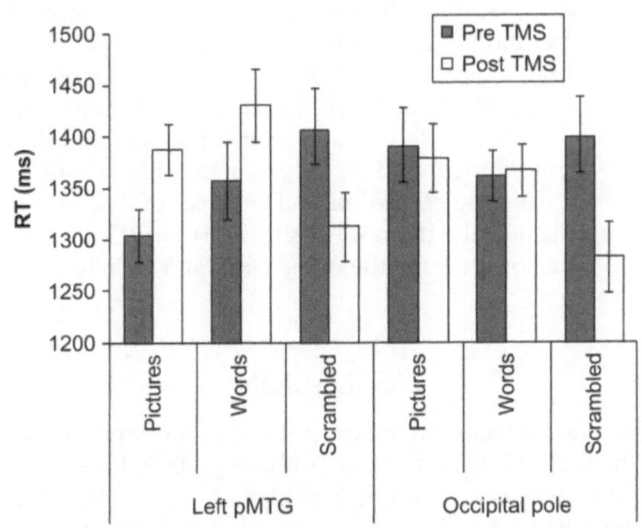

Figure 3. Reaction times before and after rTMS. Bars indicate standard error of mean, adjusted to reflect the between-condition variance used in repeated-measure designs (Loftus & Masson, 1994).

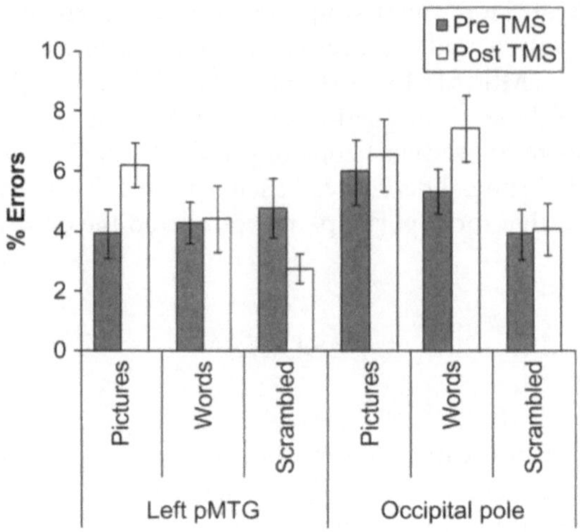

Figure 4. Error rates before and after rTMS. Bars indicate standard error of mean, adjusted to reflect the between-condition variance used in repeated-measure designs (Loftus & Masson, 1994).

reliably slowed following pMTG stimulation: Pictures: $t(13) = 2.38$, $p < .05$; Words: $t(13) = 2.49$, $p < .05$. There was no slowing on these tasks following stimulation of the occipital pole ($p > .8$).

Errors

Error rates are shown in Figure 4. A repeated-measures ANOVA was conducted with task, site and TMS (pre vs post-stimulation) as within-participants factors. This revealed a marginal main effect of task, $F(2, 26) = 3.35$, $p = .051$, and a main effect of site, $F(1, 13) = 9.05$, $p = .01$. The site effect was due to a higher error rate in the occipital pole conditions. However, there was no site × TMS interaction ($F < 1$, $p > .5$), indicating that this effect did not appear to be a consequence of stimulation. Instead this small difference could indicate uncontrolled fluctuation in participant motivation or performance across sessions. In addition, the task × TMS interaction approached significance, $F(2, 26) = 2.63$, $p = .091$. Post-hoc tests revealed that the task effect was due to a higher error rate for words than for pictures, $t(13) = 3.46$, $p < .05$; neither semantic task differed from the control task. The effect of TMS on the picture task also approached significance for the pMTG site, $t(13) = 1.97$, $p = .071$. There were no effects of TMS on error rates for the other tasks and no effects of occipital pole stimulation.

DISCUSSION

The left posterior middle temporal gyrus (pMTG) is an important area for semantic cognition (Binder et al., 2009; Cabeza & Nyberg, 2000; Indefrey & Levelt, 2004; Vigneau et al., 2006) but its function is a matter of debate. Although there is wide agreement that the region is key for *lexical*-semantic processing, it is not clear whether it also contributes to non-verbal semantic cognition. We used rTMS in healthy participants to investigate whether pMTG makes a necessary contribution to both verbal and non-verbal semantic processing. The results were unequivocal: pMTG stimulation slowed responses on verbal and non-verbal semantic tasks to an equal degree but had no such effect on difficulty-matched visual processing tasks.

These results are incompatible with the idea that pMTG is only involved in semantic processing when mapping between a word and its conceptual representation. Instead, pMTG appears to be a multimodal semantic region, necessary for both verbal and non-verbal semantic cognition. Our findings are in line with neuroimaging studies that have reported pMTG activation in purely non-verbal tasks (Kable et al., 2002; Kellenbach et al., 2003) and with neuropsychological studies that link pMTG damage with multimodal semantic deficits (Chertkow et al., 1997; Hart & Gordon, 1990; Noonan et al., 2010). Additionally, these findings may help to explain the particular pattern of deficits that occurs in Wernicke's aphasia. Wernicke's aphasia has often been characterised as a disorder of acoustic-phonological processing but it has also long been known that many patients also often have non-verbal semantic deficits (Cohen, Kelter, & Woll, 1980; De Renzi, Faglioni, Scotti, & Spinnler, 1972; Gainotti, Silveri, Villa, & Caltagirone, 1983). This has led some to propose a "dual-deficit" account in which the verbal comprehension deficit in these patients has both an acoustic-phonological component (due to damage to posterior superior temporal sulcus and gyrus) and a semantic component (due to pMTG damage; Baker, Blumstein, & Goodglass, 1981; Hickok & Poeppel, 2004). The present study confirms that pMTG makes a necessary contribution to non-verbal semantic cognition, suggesting that damage to this area is a plausible explanation for non-verbal semantic deficits in Wernicke's aphasia.

There are some limitations to the present study that should be noted. Participants were faster to perform the control task following TMS. Since this effect was observed both for pMTG and occipital pole stimulation, we interpret this as a practice effect rather than a genuine TMS effect. The mirror image matching task used as a control was unfamiliar and as such it is likely that participants improved over the course of the experiment. Such practice effects could be avoided in future studies by including a longer period of familiarisation with the task before beginning the main experiment, or by counterbalancing the order of stimulation such that some participants complete their baseline no-TMS condition after completing the TMS condition.

Moreover, although the present study highlights the multimodal role of pMTG in semantic cognition, many questions remain regarding its precise function. Some have suggested that pMTG is involved in the representation of motion or motor functions, making this region particularly important for the representation of tool and action knowledge (Campanella, D'Agostini, Skrap, & Shallice, 2010; Devlin et al., 2002; Martin, 2007; Tranel et al., 2005). Another proposal holds that this area is part of a "semantic control" network that regulates access to semantic knowledge according to the demands of the current task or context (Jefferies & Lambon Ralph, 2006; Noonan et al., 2010; Whitney, Jefferies, et al., 2011; Whitney, Kirk, et al., 2011). Either possibility is consistent with our data. The semantic association task is executively demanding because it requires a degree of problem solving to determine the relationship between probe and target. For example, when deciding whether *camel* goes with *cactus* or *rose*, overall similarity is not a good guide because camels share few features with either option. Instead, the participant must attend to one specific characteristic that camels and cacti have in common and ignore all other aspects of their semantic representations. Alternatively, the pMTG effect may have been observed because the majority of trials in the test featured manmade objects or required knowledge about how items interact (e.g., *key* with *door*; *squirrel* with *acorn*). A TMS effect would be expected if pMTG were involved in representing motions and actions associated with objects. Distinguishing between these putative functions of pMTG remains a target for future work. It is possible that different sub-regions within pMTG are involved in different elements of semantic cognition. rTMS is a particularly useful tool for investigating this possibility as it has a relatively high spatial resolution: divergent behavioural effects can be observed following stimulation to sites as little as 1 cm apart (Walsh & Rushworth, 1999).

Another challenge is to understand the interaction of the pMTG with other regions in the wider semantic neural network. Converging evidence from neuroimaging (Binney, Embleton, Jefferies, Parker, & Lambon Ralph, 2010; Devlin et al., 2000), rTMS (Pobric et al., 2007, 2010a) and from patients with semantic dementia (Bozeat et al., 2000; Mion et al., 2010) indicates that the anterior aspects of the temporal lobes are critical for representing concepts in multiple modalities. It has been suggested that anterior temporal regions act as a representational hub in which information from different sensory-motor modalities is integrated to form supra-modal conceptual representations (Lambon Ralph, Sage, Jones, & Mayberry, 2010; Patterson et al., 2007; Rogers et al., 2004). This being the case, one possibility is that the temporal lobe forms a graded representational space (Plaut, 2002) in which the most anterior parts of the temporal lobes represent supra-modal conceptual information and there is a gradual shift towards modality-specific representation in more posterior temporal regions. A representational role for action/motion properties in pMTG would fit well in such a model. Further work is needed to achieve a better understanding the function of this area, particularly regarding its structural and functional connectivity within the semantic network. In any case, the present study suggests that a full account of pMTG function must include a role in non-verbal as well as verbal comprehension.

REFERENCES

Badre, D., Poldrack, R. A., Pare-Blagoev, E. J., Insler, R. Z., & Wagner, A. D. (2005). Dissociable controlled retrieval and generalized selection mechanisms in ventrolateral prefrontal cortex. *Neuron, 47*(6), 907–918.

Badre, D., & Wagner, A. D. (2007). Left ventrolateral prefrontal cortex and the cognitive control of memory. *Neuropsychologia, 45*(13), 2883–2901.

Baker, E., Blumstein, S. E., & Goodglass, H. (1981). Interaction between phonological and semantic factors in auditory comprehension. *Neuropsychologia, 19*, 1–15.

Bedny, M., McGill, M., & Thompson-Schill, S. L. (2008). Semantic adaptation and competition during word comprehension. *Cerebral Cortex, 18*, 2574–2585.

Binder, J. R., Desai, R. H., Graves, W. W., & Conant, L. L. (2009). Where is the semantic system? A critical review and meta-analysis of 120 functional neuroimaging studies. *Cerebral Cortex, 19*, 2767–2796.

Binney, R. J., Embleton, K. V., Jefferies, E., Parker, G. J. M., & Lambon Ralph, M. A. (2010). The inferolateral aspects of the anterior temporal lobe are crucial in semantic memory: Evidence from a novel direct comparison of distortion-corrected fMRI, rTMS and semantic dementia. *Cerebral Cortex, 20*, 2728–2738.

Bozeat, S., Lambon Ralph, M. A., Patterson, K., Garrard, P., & Hodges, J. R. (2000). Non-verbal semantic impairment in semantic dementia. *Neuropsychologia, 38*(9), 1207–1215.

Cabeza, R., & Nyberg, L. (2000). Imaging cognition II: An empirical review of 275 PET and fMRI studies. *Journal of Cognitive Neuroscience, 12*, 1–47.

Campanella, F., D'Agostini, S., Skrap, M., & Shallice, T. (2010). Naming manipulable objects: Anatomy of a category specific effect in left temporal tumours. *Neuropsychologia, 48*(6), 1583–1597.

Chertkow, H., Bub, D., Deaudon, C., & Whitehead, V. (1997). On the status of object concepts in aphasia. *Brain and Language, 58*(2), 203–232.

Cohen, R., Kelter, S., & Woll, G. (1980). Analytical competence and language impairment in aphasia. *Brain and Language, 10*, 331–347.

Corbett, F., Jefferies, E., Ehsan, S., & Lambon Ralph, M. A. (2009). Different impairments of semantic cognition in semantic dementia and semantic aphasia: Evidence from the non-verbal domain. *Brain, 132*, 2593–2608.

De Renzi, E., Faglioni, P., Scotti, G., & Spinnler, H. (1972). Impairment in associating colour to form, concomitant with aphasia. *Brain, 95*, 293–304.

Devlin, J. T., Jamison, H. L., Gonnerman, L. M., & Matthews, P. M. (2006). The role of the posterior fusiform gyrus in reading. *Journal of Cognitive Neuroscience, 18*(6), 911–922.

Devlin, J. T., Moore, C. J., Mummery, C. J., Gorno-Tempini, M. L., Phillips, J. A., Noppeney, U., et al. (2002). Anatomic constraints on cognitive theories of category specificity. *NeuroImage, 15*(3), 675–685.

Devlin, J. T., Russell, R. P., Davis, M. H., Price, C. J., Wilson, J., Moss, H. E., et al. (2000). Susceptibility-induced loss of signal: Comparing PET and fMRI on a semantic task. *NeuroImage, 11*(6), 589–600.

Dronkers, N. F., Wilkins, D. P., Van Valin, R. D., Redfern, B. B., & Jaeger, J. J. (2004). Lesion analysis of the brain areas involved in language comprehension. *Cognition, 92*(1–2), 145–177.

Gainotti, G., Silveri, M. C., Villa, G., & Caltagirone, C. (1983). Drawing objects from memory in aphasia. *Brain, 106*, 613–622.

Gold, B. T., Balota, D. A., Jones, S. J., Powell, D. K., Smith, C. D., & Andersen, A. H. (2006). Dissociation of automatic and strategic lexical-semantics: Functional magnetic resonance imaging evidence for differing roles of multiple frontotemporal regions. *Journal of Neuroscience, 26*, 6523–6532.

Gough, P. M., Nobre, A. C., & Devlin, J. T. (2005). Dissociating linguistic processes in the left inferior frontal cortex with transcranial magnetic stimulation. *Journal of Neuroscience, 25*(35), 8010–8016.

Hart, J., & Gordon, B. (1990). Delineation of single-word semantic comprehension deficits in aphasia with anatomical correlation. *Annals of Neurology, 27*, 226–231.

Hickok, G., & Poeppel, D. (2004). Dorsal and ventral streams: A framework for understanding aspects of the functional anatomy of language. *Cognition, 92*(1–2), 67–99.

Hickok, G., & Poeppel, D. (2007). The cortical organization of speech processing. *Nature Reviews Neuroscience, 8*(5), 393–402.

Hilgetag, C. C., Theoret, H., & Pascual-Leone, A. (2001). Enhanced visual spatial attention ipsilateral to rTMS-induced 'virtual lesions' of human parietal cortex. *Nature Neuroscience, 4*(9), 953–957.

Holland, R., & Lambon Ralph, M. A. (2010). The anterior temporal lobe semantic hub is a part of the language neural network: Selective disruption of irregular past tense verbs by rTMS. *Cerebral Cortex, 20*(12), 2771–2775.

Howard, D., & Patterson, K. (1992). *Pyramids and Palm Trees: A test of semantic access from pictures and words*. Bury St Edmunds, UK: Thames Valley Test Company.

Indefrey, P., & Levelt, W. J. M. (2004). The spatial and temporal signatures of word production components. *Cognition, 92*(1–2), 101–144.

Jefferies, E., & Lambon Ralph, M. A. (2006). Semantic impairment in stroke aphasia vs. semantic dementia: A case-series comparison. *Brain, 129*, 2132–2147.

Kable, J. W., Lease-Spellmeyer, J., & Chatterjee, A. (2002). Neural substrates of action event knowledge. *Journal of Cognitive Neuroscience, 14*(5), 795–805.

Kellenbach, M. L., Brett, M., & Patterson, K. (2003). Actions speak louder than functions: The importance of manipulability and action in tool representation. *Journal of Cognitive Neuroscience, 15*(1), 30–46.

Kherif, F., Josse, G., & Price, C. J. (2011). Automatic top-down processing explains common left occipito-temporal responses to visual words and objects. *Cerebral Cortex, 21*(1), 103–114.

Kosslyn, S. M., Pascual-Leone, A., Felician, O., Camposano, S., Keenan, J. P., Thompson, W. L., et al. (1999). The role of Area 17 in visual imagery: Convergent evidence from PET and rTMS. *Science, 284*(5411), 167–170.

Lambon Ralph, M. A., Sage, K., Jones, R., & Mayberry, E. (2010). Coherent concepts are computed in the anterior temporal lobes. *Proceedings of the National Academy of Sciences of the United States of America, 107*, 2717–2722.

Leff, A. P., Schofield, T. M., Crinion, J. T., Seghier, M. L., Grogan, A., Green, D. W., et al. (2009). The left superior temporal gyrus is a shared substrate for auditory short-term memory and speech comprehension: Evidence from 210 patients with stroke. *Brain, 132*, 3401–3410.

Loftus, G. R., & Masson, M. E. J. (1994). Using confidence-intervals in within-subject designs. *Psychonomic Bulletin & Review, 1*(4), 476–490.

Martin, A. J. (2007). The representation of object concepts in the brain. *Annual Review of Psychology, 58*, 25–45.

Mion, M., Patterson, K., Acosta-Cabronero, J., Pengas, G., Izquierdo-Garcia, D., Hong, Y. T., et al. (2010). What the left and right fusiform gyri tell us about semantic memory. *Brain, 133*, 3256–3268.

Noonan, K. A., Jefferies, E., Corbett, F., & Lambon Ralph, M. A. (2010). Elucidating the nature of deregulated semantic cognition in semantic aphasia: Evidence for the roles of the prefrontal and temporoparietal cortices. *Journal of Cognitive Neuroscience, 22*, 1597–1613.

Noppeney, U., Phillips, J., & Price, C. (2004). The neural areas that control the retrieval and selection of semantics. *Neuropsychologia, 42*, 1269–1280.

Patterson, K., Nestor, P. J., & Rogers, T. T. (2007). Where do you know what you know? The representation of semantic knowledge in the human brain. *Nature Reviews Neuroscience, 8*(12), 976–987.

Plaut, D. C. (2002). Graded modality-specific specialisation in semantics: A computational account of optic aphasia. *Cognitive Neuropsychology, 19*(7), 603–639.

Pobric, G., Jefferies, E., & Lambon Ralph, M. A. (2007). Anterior temporal lobes mediate semantic representation: Mimicking semantic dementia by using rTMS in normal participants. *Proceedings of the National Academy of Sciences of the United States of America, 104*(50), 20137–20141.

Pobric, G., Jefferies, E., & Lambon Ralph, M. A. (2010a). Amodal semantic representations depend on both anterior temporal lobes: Evidence from repetitive transcranial magnetic stimulation. *Neuropsychologia, 48*, 1336–1342.

Pobric, G., Jefferies, E., & Lambon Ralph, M. A. (2010b). Category-specific vs. category-general semantic impairment induced by transcranial magnetic stimulation. *Current Biology, 20*, 964–968.

Price, C. J., & Friston, K. J. (2002). Degeneracy and cognitive anatomy. *Trends in Cognitive Sciences, 6*(10), 416–421.

Rodd, J. M., Davis, M. H., & Johnsrude, I. S. (2005). The neural mechanisms of speech comprehension: fMRI studies of semantic ambiguity. *Cerebral Cortex, 15*(8), 1261–1269.

Rogers, T. T., Lambon Ralph, M. A., Garrard, P., Bozeat, S., McClelland, J. L., Hodges, J. R., et al. (2004). Structure and deterioration of semantic memory: A neuropsychological and computational investigation. *Psychological Review, 111*(1), 205–235.

Saygin, A. P., Dick, F., Wilson, S. M., Dronkers, N., & Bates, E. (2003). Neural resources for processing language and environmental sounds. *Brain, 126*, 928–945.

Thompson-Schill, S. L., D'Esposito, M., Aguirre, G. K., & Farah, M. J. (1997). Role of left inferior prefrontal cortex in retrieval of semantic knowledge: A reevaluation. *Proceedings of the National Academy of Sciences of the United States of America, 94*, 14792–14797.

Tranel, D., Martin, C., Damasio, H., Grabowski, T. J., & Hichwa, R. (2005). Effects of noun–verb homonymy on the neural correlates of naming concrete entities and actions. *Brain and Language, 92*(3), 288–299.

Turken, A. U., & Dronkers, N. F. (2011). The neural architecture of the language comprehension network: Converging evidence from lesion and connectivity analyses. *Frontiers in Systems Neuroscience, 5*(1). doi:10.3389/fnsys.2011.00001.

Vigneau, M., Beaucousin, V., Hervé, P. Y., Duffau, H., Crivello, F., Houdé, O., et al. (2006). Meta-analyzing left hemisphere language areas: Phonology, semantics and sentence processing. *NeuroImage, 30*, 1414–1432.

Visser, M., Jefferies, E., Embleton, K. V., & Lambon Ralph, M. A. (2011). *Evidence for a caudo-rostral gradient of information convergence in the temporal lobes: An fMRI study of verbal and non-verbal semantic processing*. Manuscript submitted for publication.

Visser, M., Jefferies, E., & Lambon Ralph, M. A. (2010). Semantic processing in the anterior temporal lobes: A meta-analysis of the functional neuroimaging literature. *Journal of Cognitive Neuroscience, 22*, 1083–1094.

Walsh, V., & Cowey, A. (2000). Transcranial magnetic stimulation and cognitive neuroscience. *Nature Reviews Neuroscience, 1*(1), 73–79.

Walsh, V., & Rushworth, M. (1999). A primer of magnetic stimulation as a tool for neuropsychology. *Neuropsychologia, 37*, 125–135.

Whitney, C., Jefferies, E., & Kircher, T. (2011). Heterogeneity of the left temporal lobe in semantic representation and control: Priming multiple vs. single meanings of ambiguous words. *Cerebral Cortex, 21*, 831–844.

Whitney, C., Kirk, M., O'Sullivan, J., Lambon Ralph, M. A., & Jefferies, E. (2011). The neural organization of semantic control: TMS evidence for a distributed network in left inferior frontal and posterior middle temporal gyrus. *Cerebral Cortex, 21*(5), 1066–1075.

Wise, R. J. S., Scott, S. K., Blank, S. C., Mummery, C. J., Murphy, K., & Warburton, E. A. (2001). Separate neural subsystems within 'Wernicke's area'. *Brain, 124*, 83–95.

APHASIOLOGY, 2012, 26 (9), 1131–1152

Probing the involvement of the right hemisphere in language processing with online transcranial magnetic stimulation in healthy volunteers

Gesa Hartwigsen[1] and Hartwig R. Siebner[2]

[1]Language & Aphasia Laboratory, Department of Neurology, University of Leipzig, Leipzig, Germany
[2]Danish Research Centre for Magnetic Resonance, Copenhagen University Hospital Hvidovre, Hvidovre, Denmark

Background: Current models emphasize that language-related functions are predominantly organized in left-lateralized fronto-temporo-parietal cortical networks.
Aims: In this review, we summarize how "online" transcranial magnetic stimulation (TMS) during a language task can be used in healthy individuals to characterize the contribution of the stimulated area to a specific language function with a focus on the functional relevance of the right hemisphere. We first give an introduction to some basic mechanisms of TMS and outline the prerequisites for carrying out TMS studies of language. In particular, we highlight some methodological limitations and pitfalls of the TMS approach. We then review online TMS studies of language processing with a particular focus on the contribution of right hemisphere brain regions to language processing.
Main Contribution: The majority of TMS studies on language have targeted a single left-hemisphere cortical area during a language task to identify the relevance of that area for a specific aspect of language processing. TMS has also been used to characterize the involvement of homologous right hemisphere regions. These studies have provided evidence for a significant role of right hemisphere regions in different aspects of language processing, including word comprehension, reading and paralinguistic features like emotional prosody.
Conclusions: Recently, two areas have been targeted simultaneously with TMS while subjects performed a language task. This multifocal TMS approach has opened up new possibilities to compare the functional involvement of homologous regions in the right and left hemisphere and allows for the characterization of interhemispheric compensation during language processing.

Keywords: Compensation; Lesion; Lateralization; Broca; Wernicke; Speech.

Address correspondence to: Gesa Hartwigsen, Language & Aphasia Laboratory, Department of Neurology, University of Leipzig, Liebigstraße 20, 04103 Leipzig, Germany. E-mail: gesa.hartwigsen@medizin.uni-leipzig.de

GH and HRS were supported by a Grant from the "Bundesministerium fuer Bildung und Forschung" (BMBF; Grant 01GW0663), Germany. HRS was supported by a Grant of Excellence on the Control of Actions "ContAct" from the Lundbeck Foundation (R59 A5399), Denmark.

http://dx.doi.org/10.1080/02687038.2011.590573

Transcranial magnetic stimulation (TMS) is a non-invasive tool for electrical stimulation of the human cortex (Barker, Jalinous, & Freeston, 1985). The basic mechanisms of this brain stimulation technique have been covered in many recent reviews (e.g., Amassian & Maccabee, 2006; Bestmann, 2008; Sandrini, Umilta, & Rusconi, 2011; Siebner, Hartwigsen, Kassuba, & Rothwell, 2009; Ziemann et al., 2008). TMS provides a means of transiently disrupting ongoing neuronal processing in the stimulated cortex and thus permits causal conclusions to be drawn regarding the contribution of the stimulated area to a specific brain function (Paus, 2008; Walsh & Cowey, 2000). Since a single TMS pulse interferes with ongoing neural activity for several tens of milliseconds, single-pulse TMS has a sufficiently high temporal resolution to identify the time period during which the stimulated region makes a critical contribution to a given task.

At the neurobiological level the events that lead to neuronal excitation are still poorly understood. For instance, it is still largely unknown how the shape of cortical neurons and the geometric configuration of the gyrus with respect to the orientation of the TMS coil influence the efficiency of TMS. The relevance of local variations in tissue conductivity and the role of neuronal background activity for neuronal stimulation are also largely unknown.

"Online" stimulation protocols range from single or paired stimuli to the application of short high-frequency TMS bursts. Here, TMS is given during a task to disrupt ongoing neuronal processing in the stimulated area while participants perform an experimental task (e.g., Jahanshai & Rothwell, 2000; Siebner, Hartwigsen, et al., 2009). Repetitive TMS (rTMS) refers to the application of prolonged trains of stimuli, which are either given continuously as long trains at a constant rate (continuous rTMS) or intermittently as repetitive bursts (i.e., intermittent or burst-like rTMS) (e.g., Siebner & Rothwell, 2003; Ziemann et al., 2008). These rTMS protocols are usually given "offline" to induce lasting functional effects in the stimulated cortex and connected brain regions before participants perform a task (Lee, Siebner, & Bestmann, 2006). In the following we refer to rTMS for studies using repetitive *offline* TMS, while the application of short bursts of *online* TMS will be referred to as TMS.

While conventional paradigms apply uni-site TMS over a single cortical area, more recent studies have also started to include multi-site TMS over two or more areas simultaneously (Hartwigsen, Baumgaertner, et al., 2010; Hartwigsen, Price, et al., 2010). When investigating brain functions with TMS it should be borne in mind that the effects of TMS critically depend, among other factors, on the stimulation parameters, the task itself, and the time of the intervention (Siebner, Hartwigsen, et al., 2009; Siebner & Rothwell, 2003). Here we review how high-frequency TMS during language tasks (i.e., online TMS) can be used to probe the functional relevance of cortical areas in language processing in healthy individuals. For recent reviews on the investigation of language processing with TMS in aphasic patients, please refer to Devlin and Watkins (2007) or Hamilton, Medina, and Coslett (2011).

TIMING ISSUES: ONLINE VS. OFFLINE TMS

One challenge to the investigation of cognitive processes with TMS is the choice of the appropriate stimulation protocol (see Sandrini et al., 2011, for more details on the stimulation parameters). As already mentioned above, there are two different possibilities for applying TMS to investigate cognitive functions: TMS can either be applied during the task (i.e., "online") or shortly before the task (i.e., "offline"). Online TMS may consist of single pulses or short high-frequency trains given at distinct time-points during a task to perturb intrinsic neuronal activity in the stimulated area (i.e., the "virtual lesion" approach). An important advantage of TMS-induced lesions relative to studies of structural lesions is that there is insufficient time for functional reorganization to occur during online TMS and thus, the acute "lesion" effect should not be confounded by chronic processes mediating functional recovery locally and at the systems level (Walsh & Cowey, 1998, 2000).

Of note, the term "virtual lesion" implies that TMS always induces an impairment of brain functions. However, TMS-induced disruption of neuronal activity in one area may also lead to a paradoxical improvement (i.e., cognitive facilitation) in task performance. For instance, several studies reported enhanced language processing (e.g., faster reaction times) with various TMS protocols over Wernicke's area (e.g., Andoh et al., 2006; Andoh & Paus, 2011; Sparing et al., 2001; see below for details).

Although the precise mechanisms of the TMS-induced effects remain elusive, causality between a stimulated area and its involvement in a specific task function is assumed when a significant effect occurs, irrespective of whether it is facilitatory or inhibitory in nature (Sandrini et al., 2011; see also Miniussi, Ruzzoli, & Walsh, 2010).

In contrast to online TMS, offline TMS involves longer rTMS protocols that are applied shortly before participants perform an experimental task. Usually the interventional rTMS protocol is "inhibitory" (Siebner & Rothwell, 2003). This means that the rTMS intervention induces a lasting suppression of neuronal excitability in relevant areas. This conditioning approach bears some analogies to acute stroke, because inhibitory offline TMS gives rise to an acute adaptive reorganization within the non-stimulated functional loops of the networks to compensate for the TMS-induced suppression of neuronal activity in those components of the network that have been perturbed with TMS (e.g., Lee et al., 2006).

In sum, online and offline TMS represent complementary approaches: While online TMS acutely disrupts a specific function, offline TMS impairs cortical processing beyond the time of stimulation and thus can be used to induce and examine the capability of brain networks to undergo acute reorganization. Both approaches enable the researcher to investigate the functional relevance of the targeted brain area by measuring the effects of TMS on behavioural (e.g., changes in reaction times and error rates), electrophysiological (e.g., changes in the amplitude of the motor evoked potential), or neuroimaging read-outs. The latter can be done with a variety of neuroimaging techniques including positron emission tomography (PET), functional magnetic resonance imaging (fMRI), or electroencephalography (EEG).

TARGETING THE CORRECT CORTICAL AREA

Accurate placement of the TMS coil over the cortical area of interest is crucial. The motor response evoked by TMS can be used to functionally localise the primary motor cortex. A similar approach can be adopted for TMS of the visual cortex by positioning the coil at the site where TMS most reliably elicits a phosphene. In both instances TMS produces an overt response, which can be used to determine the appropriate site of stimulation. However, for most cortical areas, no such responses can be elicited. Therefore other strategies have to be used to guarantee accurate coil placement. Neuronavigated TMS based on frameless stereotaxy is the method of choice for exact coil placement and continuous monitoring of the coil throughout the TMS experiment yielding spatial accuracy in the range of a few millimetres (Denslow, Bohning, Bohning, Lomarev, & George, 2005; Herwig, Abler, et al., 2003; Neggers et al., 2004; Sack, Kohler, Linden, Goebel, & Muckli, 2006; Schonfeldt-Lecuona et al., 2005).

REMOTE EFFECTS OF TMS

An increasing body of research uses neuroimaging techniques to map TMS-evoked changes in neuronal activity throughout the brain (Siebner, Bergmann, et al., 2009). A consistent finding is that TMS gives rise to functional changes in connected cortical and subcortical areas (e.g., Bestmann, Baudewig, Siebner, Rothwell, & Frahm, 2003; Lee et al., 2003; Siebner et al., 2003).

In addition to the focal stimulation of neuronal tissue at the primary target site, TMS can influence intrinsic activity in remote brain areas because of trans-synaptic spread of excitation via cortico-cortical and cortico-subcortical projections. Using a conditioning-test paradigm, cortico-cortical interactions can be studied with TMS of two cortical motor areas (i.e., dual-site TMS). For instance, it has been shown that a conditioning TMS pulse given to one primary motor cortex can inhibit the cortico-motor excitability of the primary motor cortex in the opposite hemisphere (Di Lazzaro et al., 1999; Ferbert et al., 1992).

In sum, the effects of a TMS pulse may not only be caused by activation at the site of stimulation but may also be mediated via activation of axons projecting to remote cortical areas. Like the local effects induced in the targeted cortical area, the remote effects critically depend on the intensity of stimulation.

ADJUSTING THE STIMULATION INTENSITY TO THE SCALP-TO-CORTEX DISTANCE

When applying TMS, it should be borne in mind that the induced magnetic and electric field decreases rapidly with increasing distance from the coil. The maximal range of penetration depends on the shape and size of the coil, the employed stimulation intensity, and the responsiveness of the targeted tissue. When using a standard figure-of-eight coil, the penetration depth is sufficient to effectively stimulate the fronto-parieto-temporal language areas at the hemispherical surface. However, the distance between the stimulating coil and the cortical target region should be taken into account. The larger the distance, the higher is the intensity for effectively stimulating the targeted cortical area. At any rate, deep brain structures such as the basal ganglia, thalamus, or medial temporal lobe cannot be stimulated directly with TMS due to limited depth penetration (see Hartwigsen, Kassuba, & Siebner, 2009, for more details).

The intensity of TMS is given as percentage of maximal stimulator output (MSO) and is usually calibrated to the excitability of the primary motor hand area (M1-HAND) by using the motor threshold as reference, mainly because of a lack of more appropriate procedures. Indeed, it is unclear for which cortical areas the motor threshold of M1-HAND is a good predictor for regional excitability (Boroojerdi et al., 2002). When using the motor threshold of M1-HAND to individually adjust the intensity of stimulation, the intensity should be corrected for differences in the scalp–cortex distance between the primary motor cortex and the area that is actually targeted with TMS. As an approximation, it has been proposed to increase the stimulus intensity by 3% of MSO for every millimetre the scalp–cortex distance of the target region exceeds the scalp–cortex distance of M1-HAND (Stokes et al., 2005).

TMS STUDIES OF LANGUAGE LATERALIZATION

There have been several attempts to apply TMS in presurgical settings to non-invasively map language functions. These studies have yielded equivocal results. In a seminal study Pascual-Leone, Gates, and Dhuna (1991) tested whether TMS could serve as an alternative to the Wada test (Wada & Rasmussen, 1960) in six presurgical epilepsy patients. The authors gave short online TMS trains at rates of 8, 16, or 25 Hz over different scalp positions around the perisylvian cortex as defined by the international 10–20 electrode system in both hemispheres. A reproducible speech arrest was produced with TMS over the left but not right inferior frontal cortex 4–6 seconds after stimulation when participants counted aloud from 1. These results were in accordance with the Wada test, which revealed left hemisphere language dominance in these patients. While this study suggested that the TMS-induced speech arrest offered a non-invasive alternative for the determination of language dominance, other studies failed to replicate these promising findings and only reported complete speech arrest in some patients (e.g., Jennum et al., 1994; Micheluci et al., 1994; for review see also Hartwigsen, Siebner, & Stippich, 2010). Epstein et al. (1996) suggested that the high inter-study variability might have arisen from differences in the stimulation parameters. For instance, speech arrest was more difficult to determine at higher stimulation intensities as these intensities produced prominent muscle contractions and discomfort.

When comparing the sensitivity and specificity of pre-surgical Wada test and TMS, one should bear in mind that the Wada test affects the functions over a large region in one hemisphere for several minutes while TMS disruption is far more focal and transient. Consequently, some studies suggested that the TMS-induced effects might be too subtle to be used for preoperative evaluation of higher cognitive functions (Duzel, Hufnagel, Helmstaedter, & Elger, 1996). This may explain why the induction of speech arrest with unilateral online TMS lacks sufficient reliability in order to be clinically used for the preoperative determination of language dominance.

Knecht et al. (2002) investigated the functional relevance of lateralization of language-related brain activation. In healthy participants inter-individual differences in the degree of language lateralization were assessed with functional transcranial Doppler sonography (fTCD) and fMRI (Figure 1A). In separate sessions participants performed a picture-word verification task after offline 1Hz rTMS over left or right Wernicke's area (i.e., the left posterior superior temporal gyrus, pSTG) or an occipital control site. The rTMS-induced disruption in task performance after real rTMS correlated with both the degree and side of lateralization (Figure 1B). Participants with weak lateralization were less affected by either left hemisphere or right hemisphere TMS than participants with strong lateralization to one hemisphere. Behavioural data revealed an interaction between stimulation site and language dominance: Right-dominant participants were slower after right than left hemisphere stimulation whereas the opposite pattern was found for left-dominant participants (Figure 1C). Based on these results, it was proposed that language processing seems to be distributed evenly between both hemispheres in some participants, allowing for compensation of a unilateral brain lesion.

TMS STUDIES ON LANGUAGE PROCESSING IN THE LEFT HEMISPHERE: COMPREHENSION

Several studies investigated the functional anatomy of Broca's region in the left inferior frontal gyrus (IFG) with high-frequency online TMS (e.g., Devlin, Matthews, & Rushworth, 2003; Gough, Nobre, & Devlin, 2005; Kohler, Paus, Buckner, & Milner, 2004; Nixon, Lazarova, Hodinott-Hill, Gough, & Passingham, 2004).

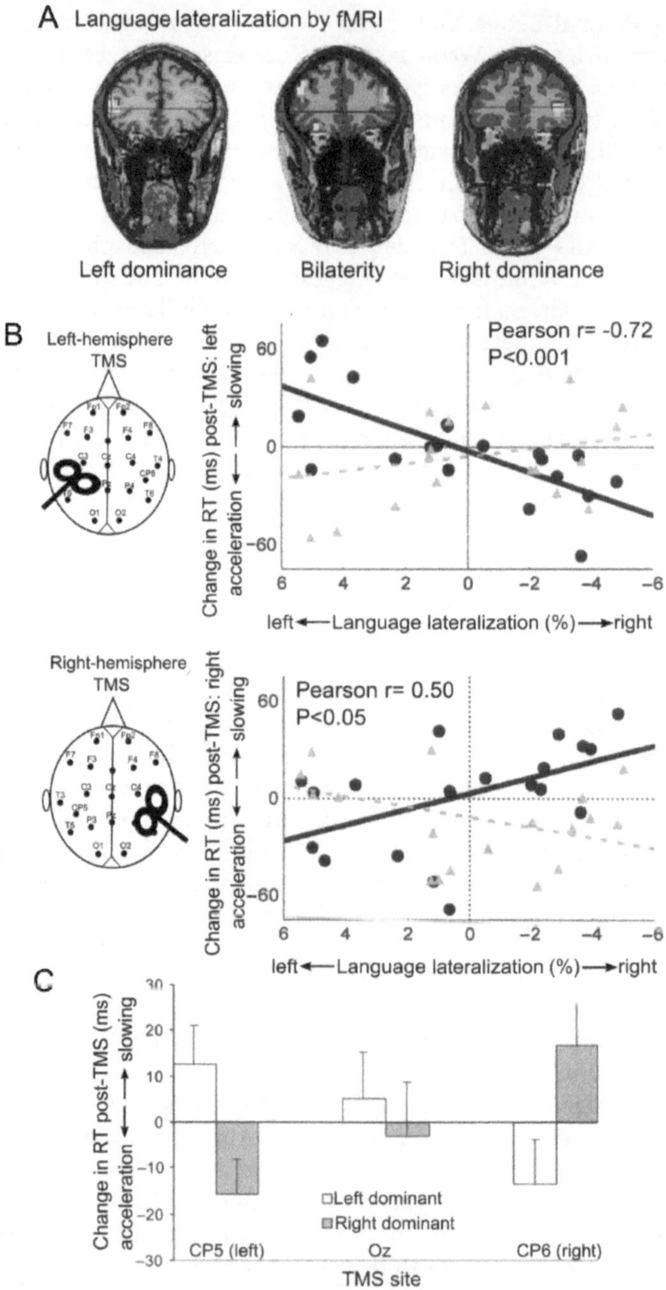

Figure 1. Correlation between the degree of language lateralization and the degree of language disruption by TMS. (A) fMRI images from participants with left, bilateral, and right language dominance (red: maximal activation). (B) x-axis: lateralization was estimated by functional transcranial Doppler sonography, y-axis: disruption of language processing (black circles). Orange triangles represent the effect of TMS on the non-linguistic control task involving matching of geometric objects. Positive values on the y-axis indicate an increase, and negative values a decrease, in response time (RT). (C) Mean changes (± SEM) in verbal processing speed assessed by response time. Interaction between left (CP5) and right (CP6) hemispheric stimulation and left ($n = 11$) and right ($n = 9$) hemispheric language dominance. Also shown are changes in RT after TMS to the midline occipital control site (Oz; $n = 6$ for left and right dominant participants, respectively). [Adapted by permission from Macmillan Publishers Ltd: Knecht et al., *Nature Neuroscience, 5*(7); 695–699. Copyright 2002.] To view this figure in colour, please see the online issue of the journal.

Together, these studies support the notion that left anterior IFG (aIFG) is necessary for semantic processing while left posterior IFG (pIFG) is more engaged in phonological processing (for more details see Devlin & Watkins, 2007) as suggested by earlier functional imaging studies (for recent reviews on neuroimaging studies see, e.g., Costafreda et al., 2006; Vigneau et al., 2006). For instance, Romero, Walsh, and Papagno (2006) investigated the neural substrates of phonological working memory. The authors found that in addition to left pIFG, the left supramarginal gyrus (SMG) of the inferior parietal cortex (IPC) also makes a critical contribution to phonological decisions in healthy volunteers: 5 Hz online TMS to either left SMG or pIFG but not to a control site significantly disrupted judgements on visually presented words in different tasks, suggesting an involvement of both regions in short term retention of verbal material as well as phonological judgements.

It should be mentioned that online TMS has also provided evidence for an involvement of the left motor cortex in speech perception (e.g., Aglioti & Pazzaglia, 2010; Aziz-Zadeh, Iacoboni, Zaidel, Wilson, & Mazziotta, 2004; Fadiga, Craighero, Buccino, & Rizzolatti, 2002; Mottonen & Watkins, 2009; Watkins & Paus, 2004; Watkins, Strafella, & Paus, 2003; for a detailed review on speech perception and the motor system see Devlin and Watkins, 2007).

TMS STUDIES ON LANGUAGE PROCESSING IN THE LEFT HEMISPHERE: PICTURE NAMING

Online TMS has also been used to investigate the role of the IFG (i.e., Broca's area) and pSTG (i.e., Wernicke's area) in picture naming. In an early study Wassermann, Cohen, Flitman, Chen, and Hallet (1996) found a stronger increase in picture-naming errors with left hemisphere 10 Hz TMS at an intensity of motor threshold compared to right hemisphere stimulation. Errors were especially prominent at left temporal sites. Flitman et al. (1998) found that 15 Hz online TMS at 120% of individual motor threshold disrupted picture-word verification when applied over left IFG. In contrast, stimulation of the homologue area in the right hemisphere or bilateral parietal cortex did not impair task performance. Using triple-pulse TMS at various time points after picture presentation onset, Schuhmann, Schiller, Goebel, and Sack (2009) further investigated the temporal dynamics of the posterior IFG in picture naming. Relative to sham stimulation, real TMS significantly increased reaction times when applied around 300 ms after picture presentation. These data confirm the essential role of the pIFG in picture naming and provide new insight into the temporal characteristics of its contribution during speech production.

Using a priming approach, other studies found facilitatory effects of single-pulse or repetitive high-frequency online TMS over left-hemispheric language areas when TMS was given immediately before picture naming (e.g., Mottaghy et al., 1999; Mottaghy, Sparing, & Topper, 2006; Sparing et al., 2001; Topper, Mottaghy, Brugmann, Noth, & Huber, 1998; Wassermann et al., 1999). In 16 healthy participants Sparing et al. (2001) compared the priming effects of high-frequency 20 Hz TMS and low-frequency 1 Hz TMS on subsequent picture naming. TMS was applied at intensities of 35%, 45% and 55% MSO over Wernicke's area, Broca's area, or the primary visual cortex. Naming latencies were decreased only immediately after 20 Hz TMS of Wernicke's area at the highest intensity. It was argued that TMS of Wernicke's area might facilitate lexical processes through a preactivation of language-related neural networks (see also Topper et al., 1998).

Together, these data provide evidence for a role of both left pIFG and left pSTG in picture naming. At the same time these studies stress the critical influence of the selected stimulation parameters (e.g., the intensity and time point of interference) on TMS-induced changes in language-related behavioural measures.

THE ROLE OF THE RIGHT HEMISPHERE IN LANGUAGE PROCESSING

A dominant role of the left hemisphere in language processing is a common notion since the days of Broca (1865) who claimed that "we speak with the left hemisphere". With his "doctrine of cerebral dominance" Dax (1865) introduced a model in which the ability of language is controlled by the cerebral hemisphere contralateral to the preferred hand. Today there is consensus about the dominance of the left hemisphere in language processing (e.g., Lindell, 2006; Shalom & Poeppel, 2008; Thiel et al., 2006) and most of the functional-anatomic models of language processing focus on the role of the left hemisphere. Knecht et al. (Knecht, Deppe, et al., 2000; Knecht, Drager, et al., 2000) demonstrated that handedness is strongly correlated with hemispheric language dominance in healthy participants. The incidence of right hemisphere language dominance was found to increase linearly with the degree of left-handedness. The authors showed that individual handedness is a predictor for hemispheric dominance in language processing. Given that right-handers are both more common and more predictably lateralised than left-handers, most studies focus on the investigation of right-handed participants. Yet the fact that the left hemisphere is the superior language processor does not necessarily imply that the right hemisphere is completely lacking linguistic ability (Lindell, 2006).

TMS STUDIES OF RIGHT HEMISPHERE CONTRIBUTIONS TO LANGUAGE PROCESSING

Although some functional imaging studies have shown right hemisphere activation in both language comprehension and production tasks in healthy participants (e.g., Ackermann & Riecker, 2004; Buchsbaum & D'Esposito, 2009; Chee, O'Craven, Bergida, Rosen, & Savoy, 1999; Devlin et al., 2003; Kemeny, Ye, Birn, & Braun, 2005; Martin, Wu, Freedman, Jackson, & Lesch, 2003; McDermott, Petersen, Watson, & Ojemann, 2003; Poldrack et al., 1999; Shibahara, 2004), there are relatively few systematic investigations on the causal role of the right hemisphere in language processing with TMS.

Contributions of the right hemisphere to language comprehension

There is a lack of studies investigating the role of the right inferior frontal cortex in semantic or phonological processing. The results of Kohler et al. (2004) may provide first evidence for a selective involvement of left but not right aIFG in episodic memory function. The authors found that 7 Hz online TMS over the left but not right aIFG enhanced the accuracy of semantic word encoding in comparison to TMS over parietal control sites. Accordingly, the authors concluded that inferior frontal TMS might have triggered a more extensive processing of the stimulated items, underlining the important role of the left aIFG but not right aIFG in episodic memory function. Recently Papagno, Fogliata, Catricala, and Miniussi (2009) investigated lexical processing of abstract and concrete nouns with online TMS. They applied 15 Hz TMS over either left IFG, left or right pSTG, left IPC or a control site in the vertex while participants decided whether a letter string represented a real word or not.

TMS selectively decreased accuracy for abstract words when applied to left pSTG, while concrete words were disrupted with TMS over right pSTG. Relative to vertex stimulation, TMS over left IFG also decreased accuracy for abstract but not concrete words while parietal TMS did not interfere with task performance. These results were taken to provide evidence for a differential involvement of both hemispheres in the storage of abstract and concrete items, with abstract lexical entries being stored in left pSTG and left IFG, and concrete items being represented in right pSTG. In contrast, the results of Lauro, Pisoni, Zerboni, and Papagno (2007) rather point towards a right hemisphere involvement of temporal cortex in the processing of abstract semantic judgements, showing that 5 Hz online TMS of the anterior inferior right but not left temporal lobe selectively interfered with abstract but not concrete semantic judgements.

Fuggetta, Rizzo, Pobric, Lavidor, and Walsh (2008) investigated the role of Wernicke's area and its right homologue in semantic processing by combining 10 Hz online TMS with event-related potentials (ERPs). In that study TMS was applied during a picture-word verification task over either left or right Wernicke's area or an occipital control site. TMS selectively increased reaction times for artifactual relative to natural items when applied over left Wernicke's area, while right hemisphere or control stimulation showed no behavioural effect. The dissociation between natural and artefactual items with TMS over Wernicke's area had a direct ERP correlate mainly reflected by systematic effects on the late positive complex over the central-parietal electrodes of the right hemisphere. This amplitude increase was taken to reflect a compensatory transfer of language function from the left to the right. It was suggested that TMS interfered with post-perceptual categorization processing of natural and artefactual stimuli that involve separate subsystems in distinct cortical areas. The absence of any TMS effect on natural items was associated with a more bilateral representation of sensory and perceptual features related to the processing of these items. The authors inferred that the interference induced by TMS over Wernicke's area might have been compensated by the functional involvement of the right hemisphere, indicating a functionally relevant integration of right hemisphere activity into the normal language network. This study stresses the value of multimodal approaches to investigate cognitive processes by combining neuroimaging techniques (here ERP recordings) with TMS.

Using a combined TMS-fMRI approach, Andoh and Paus (2011) investigated TMS-evoked changes in task-related brain activity with fMRI. In that study 10 Hz offline TMS was applied in two groups over either left or right pSTG (10 participants per group). Before and after TMS, participants performed a word recognition task using both native and foreign-language words during fMRI. The authors found increased task-related activity in the respective contralateral, non-stimulated homologue area for TMS of both hemispheres. These activity increases were interpreted in terms of adaptive short-term compensation. However, a significant decrease in reaction times for native vs foreign words was only found after TMS over left but not right pSTG. Although these results seem to support the role of the left pSTG in word recognition, it remains unclear whether the behavioural improvement was related to increased task-related activity in the contralateral right hemisphere or decreased activity at the site of stimulation (Andoh & Paus, 2011).

In two recent studies we investigated the contribution of right hemisphere areas to phonological decisions adopting a novel multifocal dual-site approach in which TMS was applied either unilaterally over homologous areas in the left or right hemisphere or simultaneously to both hemispheres (Hartwigsen, Baumgaertner, et al., 2010; Hartwigsen, Price, et al., 2010). This approach offers the possibility to study interhemispheric compensation by comparing the effects of unilateral TMS over either hemisphere with the effects of bilateral stimulation.

The first study (Hartwigsen, Baumgaertner, et al., 2010) was based on an fMRI experiment that was designed to identify modality-independent areas for phonological aspects of word comprehension (Baumgaertner, Hartwigsen, & Siebner, unpublished data). During fMRI, healthy participants made phonological judgements (i.e., does a word have two or three syllables?) or semantic judgements (i.e., does a word represent a natural or man-made item?). We found that independent of the modality used for stimulus presentation (i.e., auditory or visual), phonological as opposed to semantic processing engaged posterior brain regions, especially the supramarginal gyri (SMG) in both hemispheres (Figure 2A).

To test the functional relevance of these phonological activation patterns, we applied stereotactically guided TMS to left, right, or bilateral SMG (Figure 2B). The experimental design was comparable to our fMRI investigation (Figure 2C). Participants performed both phonological and semantic judgements and a non-linguistic perceptual control task. The latter required the participant to decide whether or not there had been a decrease in pitch towards the end of the word (auditory control task). In the perceptual visual control task, participants decided whether or not font size had decreased towards the end of the word. Mean stereotactic coordinates for right and left SMG were obtained from our fMRI investigation. The individual stimulation sites were then determined by calculating the inverse of the normalization transformation and transforming the coordinates from standard to "individual" space for each participant. During the presentation of visual or auditory words, 10 Hz TMS was randomly applied either over the left, the right or bilateral SMG (Figure 2D). This design allowed us to test for the functional relevance of right supramarginal activation during phonological decisions. We hypothesised that if right supramarginal activation is redundant to phonological processing, then reaction times or error rates would only increase when online TMS was applied over the left SMG but not the right SMG. In contrast, if the right SMG also contributes to phonological decisions, then task specific reaction times or error rates should also increase with TMS of right SMG. The simultaneous application of TMS over left and right SMG further enabled us to test whether both areas can compensate a lesion to the respective other area. We expected that if phonological decisions are possible with either the left or right SMG, the lesion effect should be greater when TMS was applied over both the left and right SMG. In contrast, if the left and right SMG are equally necessary for efficient phonological decisions, the effect of TMS should be the same irrespective of whether it was applied unilaterally or bilaterally (see Price & Friston, 2002).

The results of this study showed that TMS relative to an ineffective sham procedure significantly increased reaction times and error rates for phonological decisions but neither for the semantic nor for the perceptual task independent of the stimulated hemisphere (Figure 2E). This effect was independent of the modality used for stimulus presentation.

A control experiment revealed no effects for TMS to the neighbouring angular gyrus, indicating a high local specificity of the effect. Additionally, we tested for the sensitivity of both hemispheres to the disruptive effect of TMS. In separate blocks we

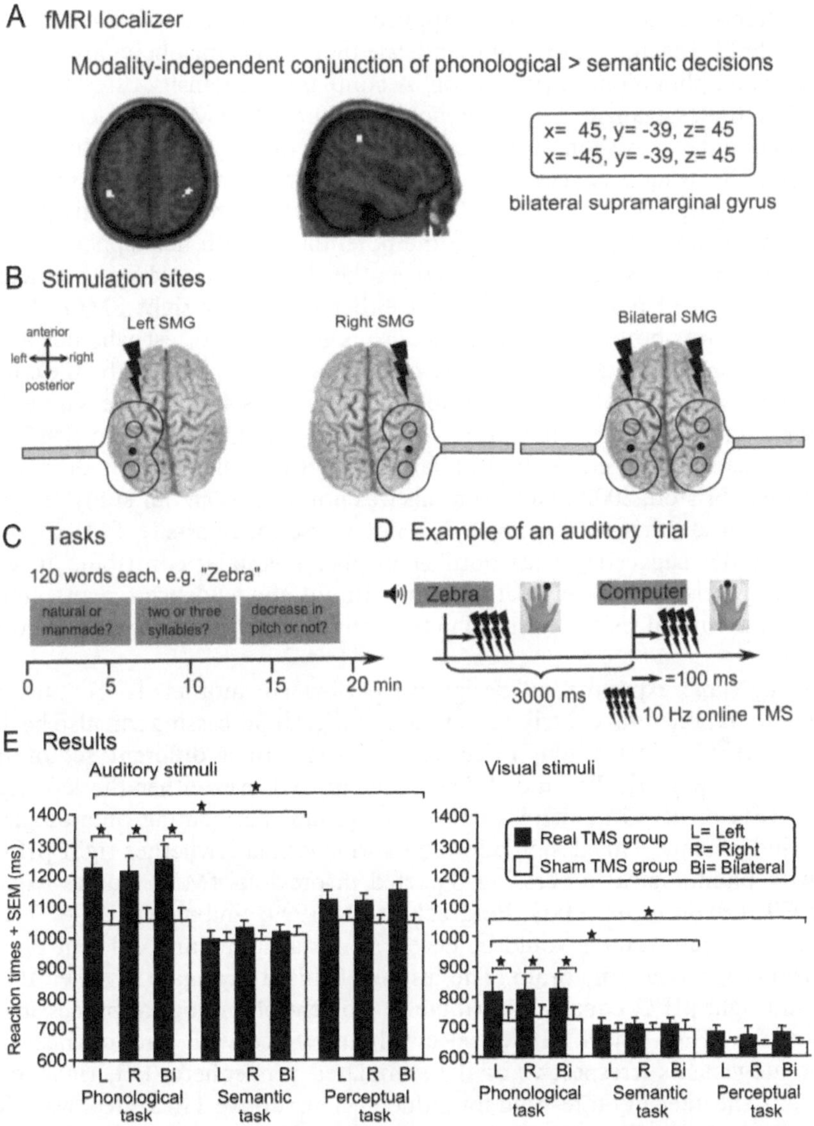

Figure 2. Effects of TMS to left and right supramarginal gyrus (SMG). (A) Stereotactic coordinates for TMS stimulation were derived from an fMRI localiser (Baumgaertner et al., unpublished data) contrasting phonological with semantic judgements. Thresholded at $p < .001$ uncorrected; see text for details. (B) Stimulation sites. (C) The three blocked tasks were presented auditorily and visually, using the same stimuli. (D) Each trial had a duration of 3.000 ms. A four-pulse train of 10 Hz TMS was applied 100 ms after word onset over left, right, or bilateral SMG. Participants responded with their left index or middle finger. (E) Effects of real vs sham TMS over left, right, and bilateral SMG. Both panels depict the significant two-way interaction between the factors task and group (i.e., real TMS selectively disrupts phonological decisions independent of the stimulated hemisphere). The three different TMS laterality sites (left, right, bilateral) and the two modalities are displayed separately for illustrating purposes, although the interaction was pooled across the factors TMS laterality site and modality. $^*p < .05$; two-tailed. [Adapted from Hartwigsen et al., *PNAS 107*(38); 16494–16499; Copyright 2010 National Academy of Sciences, USA.]

thus applied TMS with increasing intensities (55%, 60%, 75%, and 90% of individual resting motor threshold) over either left or right SMG during phonological decisions. We found an equal threshold for both hemispheres. More specifically, TMS only impaired phonological decisions when applied with an intensity of 90% of individual motor threshold. Together, the findings indicate that both hemispheres are equally necessary for intact phonological processing. A comparable intensity threshold for both hemispheres argues against an interference of right SMG TMS with left hemisphere function due to the activation of transcallosal inputs from the right to the left SMG.

Together, the results suggest that efficient modality-independent phonological judgements require both the left and the right SMG in healthy participants. Our design further enabled us to investigate the potential of both hemispheres to acutely compensate a virtual lesion of the respective other hemisphere. More specifically, the direct comparison of unilateral TMS over either the left or right SMG alone with dual-site TMS over both areas simultaneously allowed us to test whether an acute, TMS-induced unilateral "lesion effect" to one area was compensated by the contralateral, non-perturbed homologue. If phonological decisions are possible with either the left or the right pIFG, then dual-site TMS to both the left and right SMG should produce a greater lesion effect than unilateral TMS to either the left or right SMG alone (Price & Friston, 2002). However, this was not the case in our study. In contrast, our results indicate that performance was not worse for dual-site TMS as opposed to uni-site TMS, suggesting that both hemispheres equally contribute to efficient phonological decisions in the healthy brain without any evidence for an acute compensation of a "virtual lesion" induced in the homologous cortical area in the opposite hemisphere.

Using the same experimental design we performed another TMS study to test whether a similar bilateral contribution to phonological processing can also be demonstrated for pIFG (Hartwigsen, Price, et al., 2010). In a different set of healthy participants, stereotactically guided TMS was applied over either the left, right, or bilateral pIFG or aIFG (control area) in two groups performing phonological and semantic judgements. This design allowed us to investigate whether right pIFG activation with phonological processing reported in previous fMRI studies (e.g., Chee et al., 1999; Devlin et al., 2003; Poldrack et al., 1999; Shibahara, 2004; Tremblay, Monetta, & Joanette, 2004) would be necessary for accurate and efficient phonological decisions in the healthy brain. The results of this study again revealed that both the left and right pIFG equally contribute to efficient phonological processing. Thus TMS over the pIFG but not aIFG selectively interfered with phonological but not semantic judgements irrespective of the stimulated hemisphere (left, right, or bilateral). Again, the intensity threshold for inducing a disruptive TMS effect was identical for both hemispheres. These results extend previous TMS studies (e.g., Gough et al., 2005; Nixon et al., 2004; Romero et al., 2006) by demonstrating that both the left and right pIFG are equally necessary for modality-independent phonological aspects of single-word comprehension.

Together, the results of our two multifocal TMS studies challenge the notion that language processing is generally computed by the left hemisphere. At least for phonological decisions, the right and left hemisphere seem to be of similar relevance in the healthy brain. We hypothesise that a bilateral network connecting the supramarginal gyri in the IPC with the posterior inferior frontal gyri serves phonological aspects of word comprehension. Future multifocal TMS studies in healthy individuals need to address in more detail how these inferior parietal and posterior inferior frontal areas interact during phonological decision processing. Furthermore, behavioural studies of phonological processing in patients with chronic brain lesions of the right pIFG or right SMG are warranted to examine whether the left hemisphere can effectively compensate for a chronic unilateral pIFG or SMG lesion in the right hemisphere.

Contributions of the right hemisphere to reading

Early TMS-based evidence for a role of the right hemisphere in reading comes from a case study by Coslett and Monsul (1994). While acquired dyslexia has been associated with damage of the left rather than the right hemisphere since the days of Dejerine (1891, 1892), more recent studies have suggested that the right hemisphere is not "word blind" but may possess the capacity to read (e.g., Coslett & Monsul, 1994; Coslett & Saffran, 1993; Coslett, Saffran, Greenbaum, & Schwartz, 1993; Patterson, Vargha-Khadem, & Polkey, 1988). In a study by Coslett and Monsul (1994) single-pulse TMS of right but not left IPC interfered with single-word reading in a right-handed patient who had recovered from alexia caused by left hemisphere infarction. The disruptive effect of TMS was stronger for the processing of low-frequency as compared to high-frequency nouns but did not differ between stimuli of high and low imageability. Since neither left nor right hemisphere stimulation interfered with reading in three healthy control participants, it was concluded that the left hemisphere injury rendered the right IPC more vulnerable to the disruptive effects of TMS.

Braet and Humphreys (2006) found that 20 Hz online TMS over the right posterior parietal cortex (PPC) interfered with visual word recognition when healthy participants read aloud words presented either in lower case or in mIxEd-cAsE. With increasing task demands (i.e., brief presentation and low contrast), the disruptive effect of TMS was most pronounced for mIxEd-cAsE words. The authors suggested that the right parietal lobe mediates the recognition of words in unfamiliar formats by recruiting additional attentional processes.

Contributions of the right hemisphere to paralinguistic features

The right hemisphere has been implicated in more subtle aspects of language processing such as prosody, melody, emotional expression, and perception (Epstein, 1998). In accordance with this concept, brain damage to right hemisphere areas has been reported to be associated with impaired comprehension of jokes (Gardner, Ling, Flamm, & Silverman, 1975) or metaphors (Winner & Gardner, 1977). Several TMS studies also support this notion: Harpaz, Levkovitz, and Lavidor (2009) used online TMS to test whether Wernicke's area is more engaged in the processing of dominant meanings while its right homologue area processes subordinate meanings of ambiguous words. In their study participants had to make semantic decisions on ambiguous words (e.g., bank) that were followed by words associated with their dominant (e.g., teller) or subordinate (e.g., river) meanings; 10 Hz TMS was applied over left or right Wernicke's area or a control site in the vertex. Depending on the stimulated area, TMS selectively facilitated task processing of dominant or subordinate stimuli: Responses to dominant meanings were more accurate with TMS over Wernicke's area, as compared to stimulating its right homologue or the vertex. The opposite pattern emerged for subordinate meanings, with more accurate responses when TMS was given over the right homologue of Wernicke's area. This double dissociation points to a causal role of the right and left pSTG in processing subordinate and dominant meanings of ambiguous words, respectively.

Other TMS studies found right hemisphere contributions to emotional prosody discrimination (Hoekert, Bais, Kahn, & Aleman, 2008; Hoekert, Vingerhoets, & Aleman, 2010; van Rijn et al., 2005). For instance, van Rijn et al. (2005) investigated the role of the right fronto-parietal operculum in the detection of emotion in prosody with low-frequency offline rTMS. This study used two emotion discrimination tasks. In the emotional prosody task sentences of neutral content were presented and discrimination was based on the affective tone of voice. In contrast, the emotional semantic task required an affective discrimination based on the semantic content of the sentence with the tone of the voice being neutral. TMS over the right fronto-parietal operculum differentially affected reaction times for the detection of emotional prosody when compared to emotional semantics. Relative to an ineffective sham procedure, effective TMS significantly delayed the detection of withdrawal emotions (fear and sadness), but not approach emotions (happiness and anger) in the prosody condition only. Accordingly it was proposed that the right fronto-parietal operculum is crucial for the detection of withdrawal emotions in prosody. Using triple-pulse online TMS, Hoekert et al. (2008) also found a critical contribution of the right fronto-parietal operculum and the right anterior STG to emotional prosody perception. Another pilot study with nine participants by Hoekert et al. (2010) revealed increased reaction times for the classification of emotional prosody but not emotional semantics with 5 Hz online TMS over either left or right IFG compared to an ineffective sham procedure, suggesting a bilateral involvement of IFG in emotional prosody perception.

The TMS evidence for a causal involvement of right-hemispheric frontal regions in processing emotional prosody ties in with previous neuroimaging studies which have shown right-hemispheric functional activation evoked by various emotional speech comprehension tasks (e.g., Beaucousin et al., 2007; Mitchell, Elliott, Barry, Cruttenden, & Woodruff, 2003; Vingerhoets, Berckmoes, & Stroobant, 2003; Wildgruber et al., 2005). However, the precise contribution of the right vs left frontal regions and the inter-hemispheric integration of paralinguistic features remains to be determined.

Online TMS has also been used to investigate the role of the right hemisphere in metaphoric language. Pobric, Mashal, Faust, and Lavidor (2008) asked participants to perform a semantic judgement task on metaphoric expressions taken from poetry. Four types of word pairs were presented including literal word pairs (e.g., breaking glass), conventional metaphors (e.g., defence line), and novel metaphoric expressions (e.g., burning lie) as well as unrelated word pairs (e.g., bouncing coal). In a first experiment 10 Hz online TMS was applied over either right pSTS, left IFG or vertex. TMS of right pSTS disrupted processing of novel but not conventional metaphors, whereas TMS over left IFG selectively impaired processing of literal word pairs and conventional but not novel metaphors. In a second experiment TMS was applied over left or right pSTS, left or right IFG, or vertex to interfere with processing of metaphoric expressions: Again, processing of novel but not conventional metaphors was selectively disrupted by TMS over right pSTS but not by TMS of left pSTS, left IFG, or vertex. Conversely, TMS of both left and right IFG selectively impaired processing of literal word pairs and conventional but not novel metaphors. These findings are compatible with the interpretation that the right hemisphere processes a broader range of related meanings than the left hemisphere, including novel, nonsalient meanings. In addition, impaired processing of literal word pairs and conventional metaphors after both left and right IFG TMS points towards in involvement of Broca's right homologue in more salient meanings and thus more general aspects of semantic processing.

However, these results contrast with the findings of Oliveri, Romero, and Papagno (2004) who investigated the involvement of the left and right hemisphere in figurative language. In that study participants performed a sentence-to-picture matching task using opaque literal sentences (the child draws) and idiomatic phrases (he is in shape) after low-frequency 1 Hz rTMS had been applied to either left or right pSTS or IFG. In this study left hemisphere TMS disrupted task performance independent of the type of sentence, but right hemisphere TMS did not result in any impairment. The authors reasoned that sentence processing relies strictly on the left hemisphere, even in the case of opaque idiom comprehension. These partly contradictory findings may indicate that the role of the right posterior temporal cortex in metaphoric language is limited to novel metaphoric expressions while more salient meanings might be located in bilateral inferior frontal regions. While the above-mentioned studies provide causal evidence for an involvement of right hemisphere frontal and temporal areas in the processing of paralinguistic features, the precise role of these areas remains equivocal. Figure 3 summarises recent evidence for right hemisphere contributions to language processing from various studies using online TMS (see above for details).

Right hemisphere contributions to language processing: Assembling the pieces

Lesion data as well as functional imaging studies and TMS investigations in healthy volunteers provide converging evidence for a right hemisphere involvement in paralinguistic features, e.g., more subtle aspects of language processing such as (emotional) prosody, melody, emotional expression, and perception or metaphoric language (e.g., Epstein, 1998; Hoekert et al., 2010; Pobric et al., 2008; Winner & Gardner, 1977; see above for details).

Beyond paralinguistic features, there is also increasing evidence for a right hemisphere contribution to some aspects of word comprehension and reading. For

Right-hemisphere language functions indicated by online TMS

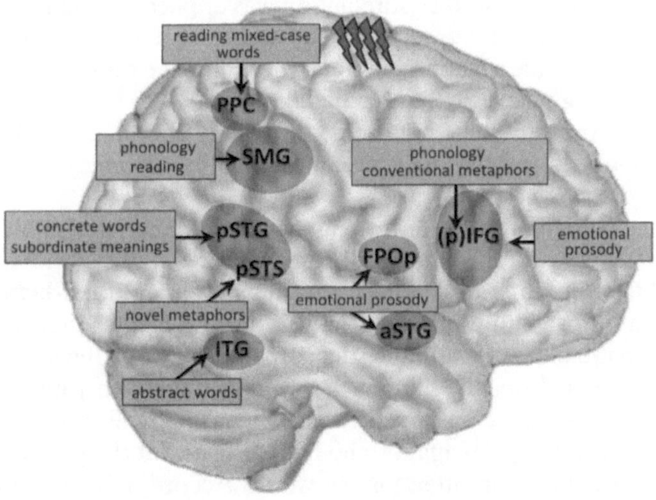

Figure 3. Illustration of right hemisphere contributions to language functions, summarising evidence from studies using different online TMS protocols (see text for details). FPOp: fronto-parietal operculum; ITG: inferior temporal gyrus; (p)IFG: posterior inferior frontal gyrus; PPC: posterior parietal cortex; SMG: supramarginal gyrus; a/pSTG: anterior/posterior superior temporal gyrus; pSTS: posterior superior temporal sulcus.

instance, a large number of functional imaging studies have shown that left as well as right hemisphere language areas of the inferior frontal cortex and parietal cortex are activated when healthy right-handed participants perform phonological tasks (Chee et al., 1999; Devlin et al., 2003; McDermott et al., 2003; Poldrack et al., 1999; Price, Moore, Humphreys, & Wise, 1997; Shibahara, 2004; Tremblay et al., 2004). In two TMS studies we investigated the functional relevance of these bilateral activation patterns (Hartwigsen, Baumgaertner, et al., 2010; Hartwigsen, Price, et al., 2010; see above). Our results demonstrated that both left and right inferior frontal and inferior parietal areas are necessary for efficient phonological decisions in healthy volunteers.

A right hemisphere contribution to phonological decisions in healthy participants may appear to be in discordance with the literature on phonological processing in patients with focal brain lesions. Damage to the right hemisphere is not typically associated with deficits in phonological processing (e.g., Dewarrat et al., 2009; Wilde 2009). While recent studies indicate that the (temporary) recruitment of homologue right hemisphere areas after left hemisphere stroke may be adaptive, longer-term language improvement is usually associated with left-hemisphere language function (Saur et al., 2006; Thiel et al., 2006; Winhuisen et al., 2005). Of note, it is still a matter of debate whether this right hemisphere activation is essential for language performance or represents "maladaptive" over-activation reflecting disinhibition rather than functioning of right-hemispheric regions due to infarction of left-hemispheric areas (e.g., Martin et al., 2004; Martin et al., 2009; Naeser et al., 2005).

Winhuisen et al. (2007) argue that restoration of the left-hemisphere network seems to be more effective for recovery after stroke, but in some cases, right hemisphere areas are integrated successfully. Likewise, Dewarrat et al. (2009) showed that word comprehension and repetition were impaired after right hemisphere damage but less frequently than after left-hemisphere damage.

How can the discrepancy between the TMS results and previous patient data be explained? One possible explanation is the difference in the time scale of functional reorganization. In our TMS studies stimulation was applied during task performance, leaving the language system no time to develop adaptive plasticity. This may be different in patients with chronic structural lesions where massive reshaping of the language network occurs during recovery (Saur et al., 2006).

In this context our results underscore the value of online TMS to investigate acute focal "lesion" effects that are not confounded by chronic processes mediating functional recovery.

A right hemisphere contribution to language processing as demonstrated by our TMS studies is in line with the findings of Raboyeau et al. (2008) who investigated the involvement of the right inferior frontal cortex in recovery after left-hemisphere stroke with PET. The authors found increased activation of the right inferior frontal gyrus in both aphasic patients and healthy participants during word retrieval following difficult re-learning. Based on this finding it was concluded that right inferior frontal activations were not a mere consequence of left-hemisphere lesions as they existed in patients as well as healthy participants who had to work out the phonetic/phonologic forms of once learned but forgotten foreign words. Accordingly, right inferior frontal activation was related to lexical retrieval following re-learning. In their study right IFG activity increased with performance improvement in aphasic patients. Although this seems to contradict studies suggesting that right hemisphere activation in chronic aphasics could be deleterious for language recovery when left frontal gyrus is not totally damaged (e.g., Buckner et al., 1996; Naeser et al., 2005b; Rosen et al., 2000),

Raboyeau et al. (2008) argue that most studies only investigated chronic word retrieval deficit processing, which is different from the dynamic lexical learning processes examined in their study. Further investigations on aphasic patients with right hemisphere lesions are necessary to understand the large literature on aphasic patients with left hemisphere damage. Here, prospective longitudinal studies might demonstrate that the right hemisphere may be more functionally relevant in the acute phase after stroke than in the chronic phase when reorganization of the language networks has occurred (Saur et al., 2006).

CONCLUSIONS AND FUTURE DIRECTIONS

Within the past few years the use of TMS in studies of language has substantially increased our knowledge about the causal role of different brain regions in various aspects of language processing. To date, however, only very few studies have systematically investigated the contribution of right hemisphere areas to language processing with TMS. These studies have started to provide evidence for a significant involvement of right hemisphere brain regions in different language functions, including phonological decisions, lexical-semantic processing, reading, (novel) metaphor processing, and emotional prosody perception. These studies vary greatly in terms of the procedure to localise the cortical target area, the selection of control sites, and the chosen experimental task, rendering direct comparison among studies difficult. The way forward is to use a multimodal approach that integrates information from different neuroimaging techniques, which will substantially increase the validity and reliability of the TMS-induced effects (Siebner, Bergmann, et al., 2009). Future studies should also consider the degree of intra- and interhemispheric interaction and compensation of different language networks. Here it would be promising to use a multifocal approach with focal "minicoils" allowing for the simultaneous application of TMS over multiple brain sites within specific language networks (e.g., Groppa et al., 2012).

REFERENCES

Ackermann, H., & Riecker, A. (2004). The contribution of the insula to motor aspects of speech production: A review and a hypothesis. *Brain and Language*, *89*, 320–328.

Aglioti, S. M., & Pazzaglia, M. (2010). Representing actions through their sound. *Experimental Brain Research*, *206*, 141–151.

Amassian, V. E., & Maccabee, P. J. (2006). Transcranial magnetic stimulation. *Conference Proceedings – IEEE Engineering in Medicine and Biology Society*, *1*, 1620–1623.

Andoh, J., Artiges, E., Pallier, C., Riviere, D., Mangin, J. F., Cachia, A., et al. (2006). Modulation of language areas with functional MR image-guided magnetic stimulation. *NeuroImage*, *29*, 619–627.

Andoh, J., & Paus, T. (2011). Combining functional neuroimaging with off-line brain stimulation: Modulation of task-related activity in language areas. *Journal of Cognitive Neuroscience*, *23*, 349–361.

Aziz-Zadeh, L., Iacoboni, M., Zaidel, E., Wilson, S., & Mazziotta, J. (2004). Left hemisphere motor facilitation in response to manual action sounds. *European Journal of Neuroscience*, *19*, 2609–2612.

Barker, A. T., Jalinous, R., & Freeston, I. L. (1985). Non-invasive magnetic stimulation of human motor cortex. *Lancet*, *1*, 1106–1107.

Beaucousin, V., Lacheret, A., Turbelin, M. R., Morel, M., Mazoyer, B., et al. (2007). FMRI study of emotional speech comprehension. *Cerebral Cortex*, *17*, 339–352.

Bestmann, S. (2008). The physiological basis of transcranial magnetic stimulation. *Trends in Cognitive Sciences*, *12*, 81–83.

Bestmann, S., Baudewig, J., Siebner, H. R., Rothwell, J. C., & Frahm, J. (2003). Subthreshold high-frequency TMS of human primary motor cortex modulates interconnected frontal motor areas as detected by interleaved fMRI-TMS. *NeuroImage*, *20*, 1685–1696.

Boroojerdi, B., Meister, I. G., Foltys, H., Sparing, R., Cohen, L. G., et al. (2002). Visual and motor cortex excitability: A transcranial magnetic stimulation study. *Clinical Neurophysiology*, *113*(9), 1501–1504.

Braet, W., & Humphreys, G. W. (2006). Case mixing and the right parietal cortex: Evidence from rTMS. *Experimental Brain Research*, *168*, 265–271.

Broca, P. (1865). Sur la faculté du langage articule. *Bulletin de la Societe d'Anthropologie de Paris*, *6*, 377–393.

Buchsbaum, B. R., & D'Esposito, M. (2009). Repetition suppression and reactivation in auditory-verbal short-term recognition memory. *Cerebral Cortex*, *19*, 1474–1485.

Buckner, R. L., Bandettini, P. A., O'Craven, K. M., Savoy, R. L., Petersen, S. E., et al. (1996). Detection of cortical activation during averaged single trials of a cognitive task using functional magnetic resonance imaging. *Proceedings of the National Academy of Sciences of the USA*, *93*, 14878–14883.

Chee, M. W., O'Craven, K. M., Bergida, R., Rosen, B. R., & Savoy, R. L. (1999). Auditory and visual word processing studied with fMRI. *Human Brain Mapping*, *7*, 15–28.

Coslett, H. B., & Monsul, N. (1994). Reading with the right hemisphere: Evidence from transcranial magnetic stimulation. *Brain and Language*, *46*, 198–211.

Coslett, H. B., & Saffran, E. M. (1993). Mechanisms of implicit reading in alexia. In M. J. Farah & G. Ratcliff (Eds.), *The neural basis of higher vision*. Pittsburgh: Carnegie-Mellon University Press.

Coslett, H. B., Saffran, E. M., Greenbaum, S., & Schwartz, H. (1993). Reading in pure alexia. The effect of strategy. *Brain*, *116*(Pt 1), 21–37.

Costafreda, S. G., Fu, C. H., Lee, L., Everitt, B., Brammer, M. J., et al. (2006). A systematic review and quantitative appraisal of fMRI studies of verbal fluency: Role of the left inferior frontal gyrus. *Human Brain Mapping*, *27*, 799–810.

Dax, M. (1865). Lesions de la moitie gauche de l'encephale coincidant avec l'oubli des signes de la pensée. *Gazette Hebdomadaire de Médecine et de Chirurgie*, *2*, 259–262.

Dejerine, J. (1891). Sur un cas de cecité verbale avec agraphie, suivi d'autopsie. *Memoires Societe Biologique*, *3*, 197–201.

Dejerine, J. (1892). Contribution a l'étude anatomoclinique et clinique des differentes variétés de cecité verbal. *CR Hebdomadaire des Sceances et Memories de la Société de Biologie*, *4*, 61–90.

Denslow, S., Bohning, D. E., Bohning, P. A., Lomarev, M. P., & George, M. S. (2005). An increased precision comparison of TMS-induced motor cortex BOLD fMRI response for image-guided versus function-guided coil placement. *Cognitive and Behavioral Neurology*, *18*, 119–126.

Devlin, J. T., Matthews, P. M., & Rushworth, M. F. (2003). Semantic processing in the left inferior prefrontal cortex: A combined functional magnetic resonance imaging and transcranial magnetic stimulation study. *Journal of Cognitive Neuroscience*, *15*, 71–84.

Devlin, J. T., & Watkins, K. E. (2007). Stimulating language: Insights from TMS. *Brain*, *130*, 610–622.

Dewarrat, G. M., Annoni, J. M., Fornari, E., Carota, A., Bogousslavsky, J., et al. (2009). Acute aphasia after right hemisphere stroke. *Journal of Neurology*, *256*, 1461–1467.

Di Lazzaro, V., Oliviero, A., Profice, P., Insola, A., Mazzone, P., et al. (1999). Direct demonstration of interhemispheric inhibition of the human motor cortex produced by transcranial magnetic stimulation. *Experimental Brain Research*, *124*, 520–524.

Duzel, E., Hufnagel, A., Helmstaedter, C., & Elger, C. (1996). Verbal working memory components can be selectively influenced by transcranial magnetic stimulation in patients with left temporal lobe epilepsy. *Neuropsychologia*, *34*, 775–783.

Epstein, C. M. (1998). Transcranial magnetic stimulation: Language function. *Journal of Clinical Neurophysiology*, *15*, 325–332.

Epstein, C. M., Lah, J. J., Meador, K., Weissman, J. D., Gaitan, L. E., et al. (1996). Optimum stimulus parameters for lateralised suppression of speech with magnetic brain stimulation. *Neurology*, *47*, 1590–1593.

Fadiga, L., Craighero, L., Buccino, G., & Rizzolatti, G. (2002). Speech listening specifically modulates the excitability of tongue muscles: A TMS study. *European Journal of Neuroscience*, *15*, 399–402.

Ferbert, A., Priori, A., Rothwell, J. C., Day, B. L., Colebatch, J. G., et al. (1992). Interhemispheric inhibition of the human motor cortex. *Journal of Physiology*, *453*, 525–546.

Flitman, S. S., Grafman, J., Wassermann, E. M., Cooper, V., O'Grady, J., et al. (1998). Linguistic processing during repetitive transcranial magnetic stimulation. *Neurology*, *50*, 175–181.

Fuggetta, G., Rizzo, S., Pobric, G., Lavidor, M., & Walsh, V. (2008). Functional representation of living and nonliving domains across the cerebral hemispheres: A combined event-related potential/transcranial magnetic stimulation study. *Journal of Cognitive Neuroscience*, *21*(2), 403–414.

Gardner, H., Ling, P. K., Flamm, L., & Silverman, J. (1975). Comprehension and appreciation of humorous material following brain damage. *Brain*, *98*, 399–412.

Gough, P. M., Nobre, A. C., & Devlin, J. T. (2005). Dissociating linguistic processes in the left inferior frontal cortex with transcranial magnetic stimulation. *Journal of Neuroscience*, *25*, 8010–8016.

Groppa, S., Schlaak, B. H., Münchau, A., Werner-Petroll, N., Dünnweber, J., Bäumer, T., . . . Siebner, H. R. (2012). The human dorsal premotor cortex facilitates the excitability of ipsilateral primary motor cortex via a short latency cortico-cortical route. *Human Brain Mapping*, *33*, 419–430.

Hamilton, R. H., Medina, J., & Coslett, H. B. (2011). Anatomic specificity of enhanced naming in patients with chronic nonfluent aphasia using transcranial magnetic stimulation. *Aphasiology*, forthcoming.

Harpaz, Y., Levkovitz, Y., & Lavidor, M. (2009). Lexical ambiguity resolution in Wernicke's area and its right homologue. *Cortex*, *45*, 1097–1103.

Hartwigsen, G., Baumgaertner, A., Price, C. J., Koehnke, M., Ulmer, S., et al. (2010). Phonological decisions require both the left and right supramarginal gyri. *Proceedings of the National Academy of Sciences of the USA*, *107*, 16494–16499.

Hartwigsen, G., Kassuba, T., & Siebner, H. R. (2009) Combining transcranial magnetic stimulation with (f)MRI. In S. Ulmer & O. Jansen (Eds.), *fMRI: Basics and clinical applications* (pp. 155–167). Heidelberg: Springer.

Hartwigsen, G., Price, C. J., Baumgaertner, A., Geiss, G., Koehnke, M., et al. (2010). The right posterior inferior frontal gyrus contributes to phonological word decisions in the healthy brain: Evidence from dual-site TMS. *Neuropsychologia*, *48*, 3155–3163.

Hartwigsen, G., Siebner, H. R., & Stippich, C. (2010). Preoperative functional magnetic resonance imaging (fMRI) and transcranial magnetic stimulation (TMS). *Current Medical Imaging Reviews*, *6*(4), 220–231.

Herwig, U., Abler, B., Schonfeldt-Lecuona, C., Wunderlich, A., Grothe, J., et al. (2003a). Verbal storage in a premotor-parietal network: Evidence from fMRI-guided magnetic stimulation. *NeuroImage*, *20*, 1032–1041.

Herwig, U., Satrapi, P., & Schonfeldt-Lecuona, C. (2003b). Using the international 10–20 EEG system for positioning of transcranial magnetic stimulation. *Brain Topography*, *16*, 95–99.

Hoekert, M., Bais, L., Kahn, R. S., & Aleman, A. (2008). Time course of the involvement of the right anterior superior temporal gyrus and the right fronto-parietal operculum in emotional prosody perception. *PlosOne*, *3*(5), e2244.

Hoekert, M., Vingerhoets, G., & Aleman, A. (2010). Results of a pilot study on the involvement of bilateral inferior frontal gyri in emotional prosody perception: An rTMS study. *BMC Neuroscience*, *11*, 93.

Jahanshahi, M., & Rothwell, J. (2000). Transcranial magnetic stimulation studies of cognition: An emerging field. *Experimental Brain Research*, *131*(1), 1–9.

Jennum, P., Friberg, L., Fuglsang-Frederiksen, A., & Dam, M. (1994). Speech localisation using repetitive transcranial magnetic stimulation. *Neurology*, *44*, 269–273.

Kemeny, S., Ye, F. Q., Birn, R., & Braun, A. R. (2005). Comparison of continuous overt speech fMRI using BOLD and arterial spin labeling. *Human Brain Mapping*, *24*, 173–183.

Knecht, S., Deppe, M., Drager, B., Bobe, L., Lohmann, H., et al. (2000). Language lateralisation in healthy right-handers. *Brain*, *123*(Pt 1), 74–81.

Knecht, S., Drager, B., Deppe, M., Bobe, L., Lohmann, H., et al. (2000). Handedness and hemispheric language dominance in healthy humans. *Brain*, *123*(Pt 12), 2512–2518.

Knecht, S., Floel, A., Drager, B., Breitenstein, C., Sommer, J., et al. (2002). Degree of language lateralisation determines susceptibility to unilateral brain lesions. *Nature Neuroscience*, *5*, 695–699.

Kohler, S., Paus, T., Buckner, R. L., & Milner, B. (2004). Effects of left inferior prefrontal stimulation on episodic memory formation: A two-stage fMRI-rTMS study. *Journal of Cognitive Neuroscience*, *16*, 178–188.

Lauro, L. J., Pisoni, A., Zerboni, H., & Papagno, C. (2007). The neural correlates of abstract versus concrete words: Evidence from an rTMS study. *Brain and Language*, *103*, 146–147.

Lee, L., Siebner, H., & Bestmann, S. (2006). Rapid modulation of distributed brain activity by transcranial magnetic stimulation of human motor cortex. *Behavioral Neurology*, *17*(3–4), 135–148.

Lee, L., Siebner, H. R., Rowe, J. B., Rizzo, V., Rothwell, J. C., et al. (2003). Acute remapping within the motor system induced by low-frequency repetitive transcranial magnetic stimulation. *Journal of Neuroscience*, *23*, 5308–5318.

Lindell, A. K. (2006). In your right mind: Right hemisphere contributions to language processing and production. *Neuropsychological Reviews*, *16*, 131–148.

Martin, P. I., Naeser, M. A., Ho, M., Doron, K. W., Kurland, J., et al. (2009). Overt naming fMRI pre- and post-TMS: Two nonfluent aphasia patients, with and without improved naming post-TMS. *Brain and Language*, *111*(1), 20–35.

Martin, P. I., Naeser, M. A., Theoret, H., Tormos, J. M., Nicholas, M., et al. (2004). Transcranial magnetic stimulation as a complementary treatment for aphasia. *Seminars in Speech and Language*, *25*, 181–191.

Martin, R. C., Wu, D., Freedman, M., Jackson, E. F., & Lesch, M. (2003). An event-related fMRI investigation of phonological versus semantic short-term memory. *Journal of Neurolinguistics*, *16*, 341–360.

McDermott, K. B., Petersen, S. E., Watson, J. M., & Ojemann, J. G. (2003). A procedure for identifying regions preferentially activated by attention to semantic and phonological relations using functional magnetic resonance imaging. *Neuropsychologia*, *41*, 293–303.

Michelucci, R., Valzania, F., Passarelli, D., Santangelo, M., Rizzi, R., et al. (1994). Rapid-rate transcranial magnetic stimulation and hemispheric language dominance: Usefulness and safety in epilepsy. *Neurology*, *44*, 1697–1700.

Miniussi, C., Ruzzoli, M., & Walsh, V. (2010). The mechanism of transcranial magnetic stimulation in cognition. *Cortex*, *46*, 128–130.

Mitchell, R. L., Elliott, R., Barry, M., Cruttenden, A., & Woodruff, P. W. (2003). The neural response to emotional prosody, as revealed by functional magnetic resonance imaging. *Neuropsychologia*, *41*, 1410–1421.

Mottaghy, F. M., Hungs, M., Brugmann, M., Sparing, R., Boroojerdi, B., et al. (1999). Facilitation of picture naming after repetitive transcranial magnetic stimulation. *Neurology*, *53*, 1806–1812.

Mottaghy, F. M., Sparing, R., & Topper, R. (2006). Enhancing picture naming with transcranial magnetic stimulation. *Behavioral Neurology*, *17*, 177–186.

Mottonen, R., & Watkins, K. E. (2009). Motor representations of articulators contribute to categorical perception of speech sounds. *Journal of Neuroscience*, *29*, 9819–9825.

Naeser, M. A., Martin, P. I., Nicholas, M., Baker, E. H., Seekins, H., et al. (2005a). Improved naming after TMS treatments in a chronic, global aphasia patient-case report. *Neurocase*, *11*, 182–193.

Naeser, M. A., Martin, P. I., Nicholas, M., Baker, E. H., Seekins, H., et al. (2005b). Improved picture naming in chronic aphasia after TMS to part of right Broca's area: An open-protocol study. *Brain and Language*, *93*, 95–105.

Neggers, S. F., Langerak, T. R., Schutter, D. J., Mandl, R. C., Ramsey, N. F., et al. (2004). A stereotactic method for image-guided transcranial magnetic stimulation validated with fMRI and motor-evoked potentials. *NeuroImage*, *21*, 1805–1817.

Nixon, P., Lazarova, J., Hodinott-Hill, I., Gough, P., & Passingham, R. (2004). The inferior frontal gyrus and phonological processing: An investigation using rTMS. *Journal of Cognitive Neuroscience*, *16*, 289–300.

Oliveri, M., Romero, L., & Papagno, C. (2004). Left but not right temporal involvement in opaque idiom comprehension: A repetitive transcranial magnetic stimulation study. *Journal of Cognitive Neuroscience*, *16*, 848–855.

Papagno, C., Fogliata, A., Catricala, E., & Miniussi, C. (2009). The lexical processing of abstract and concrete nouns. *Brain Research*, *1263*, 78–86.

Pascual-Leone, A., Gates, J. R., & Dhuna, A. (1991). Induction of speech arrest and counting errors with rapid-rate transcranial magnetic stimulation. *Neurology*, *41*, 697–702.

Patterson, D., Vargha-Khadem, F., & Polkey, C. (1988). Reading with one hemisphere. *Brain*, *112*, 39–63.

Paus, T. (2008). Combining brain imaging with brain stimulation: Causality and connectivity. In E. M. Wassermann, C. M. Epstein, U. Ziemann, V. Walsh, T. Paus, & S. H. Lisanby (Eds.), *The Oxford handbook of transcranial stimulation* (pp. 539–547). New York: Oxford University Press.

Pobric, G., Mashal, N., Faust, M., & Lavidor, M. (2008). The role of the right cerebral hemisphere in processing novel metaphoric expressions: A transcranial magnetic stimulation study. *Journal of Cognitive Neuroscience*, *20*, 170–181.

Poldrack, R. A., Wagner, A. D., Prull, M. W., Desmond, J. E., Glover, G. H., et al. (1999). Functional specialization for semantic and phonological processing in the left inferior prefrontal cortex. *NeuroImage*, *10*, 15–35.

Price, C. J., & Friston, K. J. (2002). Degeneracy and cognitive anatomy. *Trends in Cognitive Sciences*, *6*, 416–421.

Price, C. J., Moore, C. J., Humphreys, G. W., & Wise, R. J. S. (1997). Segregating semantic from phonological processes during reading. *Journal of Cognitive Neuroscience*, *9*(6), 727–733.

Raboyeau, G., De Boissezon, X., Marie, N., Balduyck, S., Puel, M., et al. (2008). Right hemisphere activation in recovery from aphasia: Lesion effect or function recruitment? *Neurology*, *70*, 290–298.

Romero, L., Walsh, V., & Papagno, C. (2006). The neural correlates of phonological short-term memory: A repetitive transcranial magnetic stimulation study. *Journal of Cognitive Neuroscience*, *18*, 1147–1155.

Rosen, H. J., Petersen, S. E., Linenweber, M. R., Snyder, A. Z., White, D. A., et al. (2000). Neural correlates of recovery from aphasia after damage to left inferior frontal cortex. *Neurology*, *55*, 1883–1894.

Sack, A. T., Cohen Kadosh, R., Schuhmann, T., Moerel, M., Walsh, V., et al. (2009). Optimizing functional accuracy of TMS in cognitive studies: A comparison of methods. *Journal of Cognitive Neuroscience*, *21*, 207–221.

Sack, A. T., Kohler, A., Linden, D. E., Goebel, R., & Muckli, L. (2006). The temporal characteristics of motion processing in hMT/V5+: Combining fMRI and neuronavigated TMS. *NeuroImage*, *29*, 1326–1335.

Saur, D., Lange, R., Baumgaertner, A., Schraknepper, V., Willmes, K., et al. (2006). Dynamics of language reorganisation after stroke. *Brain*, *129*, 1371–1384.

Sandrini, M., Umilta, C., & Rusconi, E. (2011). The use of transcranial magnetic stimulation in cognitive neuroscience: A new synthesis of methodological issues. *Neuroscience and Biobehavioral Reviews*, *35*, 516–536.

Schonfeldt-Lecuona, C., Thielscher, A., Freudenmann, R. W., Kron, M., Spitzer, M., et al. (2005). Accuracy of stereotaxic positioning of transcranial magnetic stimulation. *Brain Topography*, *17*, 253–259.

Schuhmann, T., Schiller, N. O., Goebel, R., & Sack, A. T. (2009). The temporal characteristics of functional activation in Broca's area during overt picture naming. *Cortex*, *45*, 1111–1116.

Shalom, D. B., & Poeppel, D. (2008). Functional anatomic models of language: Assembling the pieces. *Neuroscientist*, *14*, 119–127.

Shibahara, N. (2004). Picture-name priming in the cerebral hemispheres: Evidence for phonological access in the right hemisphere. *Perceptual and Motor Skills*, *99*, 305–314.

Siebner, H. R., Bergmann, T. O., Bestmann, S., Massimini, M., Johansen-Berg, H., et al. (2009). Consensus paper: Combining transcranial stimulation with neuroimaging. *Brain Stimulation*, *2*, 58–80.

Siebner, H. R., Filipovic, S. R., Rowe, J. B., Cordivari, C., Gerschlager, W., et al. (2003). Patients with focal arm dystonia have increased sensitivity to slow-frequency repetitive TMS of the dorsal premotor cortex. *Brain*, *126*, 2710–2725.

Siebner, H. R., Hartwigsen, G., Kassuba, T., & Rothwell, J. C. (2009). How does transcranial magnetic stimulation modify neuronal activity in the brain? Implications for studies of cognition. *Cortex*, *45*, 1035–1042.

Siebner, H. R., & Rothwell, J. (2003). Transcranial magnetic stimulation: New insights into representational cortical plasticity. *Experimental Brain Research*, *148*, 1–16.

Sparing, R., Buelte, D., Meister, I. G., Paus, T., & Fink, G. R. (2008). Transcranial magnetic stimulation and the challenge of coil placement: A comparison of conventional and stereotaxic neuronavigational strategies. *Human Brain Mapping*, *29*, 82–96.

Sparing, R., Mottaghy, F. M., Hungs, M., Brugmann, M., Foltys, H., et al. (2001). Repetitive transcranial magnetic stimulation effects on language function depend on the stimulation parameters. *Journal of Clinical Neurophysiology*, *18*, 326–330.

Stokes, M. G., Chambers, C. D., Gould, I. C., Henderson, T. R., Janko, N. E., et al. (2005). Simple metric for scaling motor threshold based on scalp-cortex distance: Application to studies using transcranial magnetic stimulation. *Journal of Neurophysiology*, *94*, 4520–4527.

Thiel, A., Habedank, B., Herholz, K., Kessler, J., Winhuisen, L., et al. (2006). From the left to the right: How the brain compensates progressive loss of language function. *Brain and Language*, *98*, 57–65.

Topper, R., Mottaghy, F. M., Brugmann, M., Noth, J., & Huber, W. (1998). Facilitation of picture naming by focal transcranial magnetic stimulation of Wernicke's area. *Experimental Brain Research*, *121*, 371–378.

Tremblay, T., Monetta, L., & Joanette, Y. (2004). Phonological processing of words in right- and left-handers. *Brain and Cognition*, *55*, 427–432.

van Rijn, S., Aleman, A., van Diessen, E., Berckmoes, C., Vingerhoets, G., et al. (2005). What is said or how it is said makes a difference: Role of the right fronto-parietal operculum in emotional prosody as revealed by repetitive TMS. *European Journal of Neuroscience*, *21*, 3195–3200.

Vigneau, M., Beaucousin, V., Herve, P. Y., Duffau, H., Crivello, F., et al. (2006). Meta-analyzing left hemisphere language areas: Phonology, semantics, and sentence processing. *NeuroImage*, *30*, 1414–1432.

Vingerhoets, G., Berckmoes, C., & Stroobant, N. (2003). Cerebral hemodynamics during discrimination of prosodic and semantic emotion in speech studied by transcranial doppler ultrasonography. *Neuropsychology*, *17*, 93–99.

Wada, J., & Rasmussen, T. (1960). Intracarotid injection of sodium amytal for the lateralisation of cerebral speech dominance: Experimental and clinical obserations. *Journal of Neurosurgery*, *17*, 266–282.

Walsh, V., & Cowey, A. (1998). Magnetic stimulation studies of visual cognition. *Trends in Cognitive Sciences*, *2*, 103–110.

Walsh, V., & Cowey, A. (2000). Transcranial magnetic stimulation and cognitive neuroscience. *Nature Reviews in Neuroscience*, *1*, 73–79.

Wassermann, E. M., Blaxton, T. A., Hoffman, E. A., Berry, C. D., Oletsky, H., et al. (1999). Repetitive transcranial magnetic stimulation of the dominant hemisphere can disrupt visual naming in temporal lobe epilepsy patients. *Neuropsychologia*, *37*, 537–544.

Wassermann, E. M., Cohen, L. G., Flitman, S. S., Chen, R., & Hallett, M. (1996). Seizures in healthy people with repeated "safe" trains of transcranial magnetic stimuli. *Lancet*, *347*, 825–826.

Watkins, K., & Paus, T. (2004). Modulation of motor excitability during speech perception: The role of Broca's area. *Journal of Cognitive Neuroscience*, *16*, 978–987.

Watkins, K. E., Strafella, A. P., & Paus, T. (2003). Seeing and hearing speech excites the motor system involved in speech production. *Neuropsychologia*, *41*, 989–994.

Wilde, M. C. (2009). Lesion location and repeatable battery for the assessment of neuropsychological status performance in acute ischemic stroke. *The Clinical Neuropsychologist*, *23*, 1744–4144.

Wildgruber, D., Riecker, A., Hertrich, I., Erb, M., Grodd, W., et al. (2005). Identification of emotional intonation evaluated by fMRI. *NeuroImage*, *24*, 1233–1241.

Winhuisen, L., Thiel, A., Schumacher, B., Kessler, J., Rudolf, J., et al. (2005). Role of the contralateral inferior frontal gyrus in recovery of language function in poststroke aphasia: A combined repetitive transcranial magnetic stimulation and positron emission tomography study. *Stroke*, *36*, 1759–1763.

Winhuisen, L., Thiel, A., Schumacher, B., Kessler, J., Rudolf, J., et al. (2007). The right inferior frontal gyrus and poststroke aphasia: A follow-up investigation. *Stroke*, *38*, 1286–1292.

Winner, E., & Gardner, H. (1977). The comprehension of metaphor in brain-damaged patients. *Brain*, *100*, 717–729.

Ziemann, U., Paulus, W., Nitsche, M. A., Pascual-Leone, A., Byblow, W. D., et al. (2008). Consensus: Motor cortex plasticity protocols. *Brain Stimulation*, *1*, 164–182.

APHASIOLOGY, 2012, 26 (9), 1153–1168

Finding the right words: Transcranial magnetic stimulation improves discourse productivity in non-fluent aphasia after stroke

Jared Medina[1], Catherine Norise[2], Olufunsho Faseyitan[1], H. Branch Coslett[1], Peter E. Turkeltaub[2], and Roy H. Hamilton[1]

[1]Department of Neurology, University of Pennsylvania, Philadelphia, PA, USA
[2]Department of Neurology, Georgetown University, Washington, DC, USA

Background: Loss of fluency is a significant source of functional impairment in many individuals with aphasia. Repetitive transcranial magnetic stimulation (rTMS) administered to the right inferior frontal gyrus (IFG) has been shown to facilitate naming in persons with chronic left hemisphere stroke and non-fluent aphasia. However, changes in fluency in aphasic participants receiving rTMS have not been adequately explored.
Aims: To determine whether rTMS improves fluency in individuals with chronic nonfluent aphasia, and to identify aspects of fluency that are modulated in persons who respond to rTMS.
Methods & Procedures: Ten individuals with left hemisphere MCA strokes and mild to moderate non-fluent aphasia participated in the study. Before treatment participants were asked to describe the Cookie Theft picture in three separate sessions. During treatment all participants received 1200 pulses of 1 Hz rTMS daily in 10 sessions over 2 weeks at a site that had previously been shown to improve naming. Participants repeated the Cookie Theft description 2 months after treatment. Five participants initially received sham stimulation instead of real TMS; 2 months after sham treatment these individuals received real rTMS. Performance both at baseline and after stimulation was coded using Quantitative Production Analysis (Saffran, Berndt, & Schwartz, 1989) and Correct Information Unit (Nicholas & Brookshire, 1993) analysis.
Outcomes & Results: Across all participants ($n = 10$), real rTMS treatment resulted in a significant increase in multiple measures of discourse productivity compared to baseline performance. There was no significant increase in measures of sentence productivity or grammatical accuracy. There was no significant increase from baseline in the sham condition ($n = 5$) on any study measures.
Conclusions: Stimulation of the right IFG in patients with chronic non-fluent aphasia facilitates discourse production. We posit that this effect may be attributable to improved lexical-semantic access.

Keywords: Language; Aphasia; Transcranial magnetic stimulation; TMS; Pars triangularis; Fluency; Neurorehabilitation.

Address correspondence to: Roy H. Hamilton, MD, MS, Goddard Laboratories, Room 518, University of Pennsylvania, 3710 Hamilton Walk, Philadelphia, PA 19104, USA. E-mail: Roy.Hamilton@uphs.upenn.edu

Sources of funding: HBC: NIH 2R01 DC05672-04A2. RHH: NIH/NINDS 1K01NS060995-01A1. RHH: Robert Wood Johnson Foundation/Harold Amos Medical Faculty Development Program. PET: American Academy of Neurology Foundation.

http://dx.doi.org/10.1080/02687038.2012.710316

Failure of spontaneously generated fluent speech is a source of considerable disability for many individuals with aphasia after stroke, particularly those with anterior lesions of the left hemisphere. Nonfluent aphasia is typically characterised by difficulties in speech output, with deficits including interrupted speech, word omission, loss or misuse of inflectional morphology, and utterances with limited syntactic complexity. However, depending on lesion size and location, different individuals may experience a variety of specific impairments to varying degrees, including but not limited to deficits in speech initiation, poor retrieval of accurate semantic or lexical representations, disrupted sequencing of articulatory movements, or inaccurate grammatical constructions (Gleason, Goodglass, Green, Ackerman, & Hyde, 1975; Kolk & Heeschen, 1990).

Recent studies have suggested that exogenous manipulation of cortical activity with repetitive transcranial magnetic stimulation (rTMS) may improve naming in persons with chronic left hemisphere stroke and nonfluent aphasia (e.g., Barwood et al., 2011; Martin et al., 2009; Naeser et al., 2005; Weiduchat et al., 2011; and others). Most investigations in this area have employed low-frequency (1 Hz) inhibitory rTMS of the right inferior frontal gyrus (RIFG), and within that region many studies have focused on the right pars triangularis (RPTr). The specific mechanisms by which rTMS administered to this region produces beneficial changes in language ability are debated. Proposed mechanisms have included the dampening of inhibitory transcallosal connections between the right and left hemispheres or modification of intrahemispheric connections within a compensatory network of right hemisphere language areas (see Hamilton, Chrysikou, & Coslett, 2011 for a review of this topic).

To date most studies investigating the effects of rTMS on language recovery in patients with chronic nonfluent aphasia have focused on changes in naming ability. Naeser and colleagues (2005) reported improved performance on the Boston Naming Test and naming subtests of the Boston Diagnostic Aphasia Examination in four participants who received 1 Hz rTMS to the RIFG for 10 days (see also Barwood et al., 2011; Hamilton et al., 2010; Martin et al., 2009). Investigators have used transient changes in naming ability after single sessions of 1 Hz rTMS as a strategy for identifying optimal stimulation targets within right inferior frontal gyrus in nonfluent aphasic individuals (Hamilton et al., 2010; Naeser et al., 2011; Turkeltaub, Coslett, et al., 2011).

Despite the impact of dysfluency on the functional abilities of many individuals with nonfluent aphasia, relatively little has been reported with regard to the effect of right hemisphere rTMS on this aspect of language. To date only three studies have reported spontaneous speech data in individuals who have undergone right hemisphere rTMS treatment. These studies have reported the greatest number of words in a phrase (Barwood et al., 2011; Martin et al., 2009; Naeser et al., 2005), articulatory agility (Naeser et al., 2005), or picture description complexity index (Barwood et al., 2011) as dependent variables. However, detailed coding schemes, like Quantitative Production Analysis (QPA; Rochon, Saffran, Berndt, & Schwartz, 2000; Saffran et al., 1989), can be used to fully characterise the various dissociable aspects of language production that contribute to fluent spontaneous speech. After coding spontaneous speech, past experimenters have found that specific variables in speech production in aphasics tend to correlate. For example, Rochon and colleagues (2000) found that a three-factor model (sentence structure, unbound morpheme frequency, speech rate) characterised performance in a set of 37 aphasic individuals. Others have grouped measures from QPA into categories based on various aspects of language (Gordon, 2006).

We examined whether right IFG rTMS treatment changed narrative speech production in a group of nonfluent aphasic participants using QPA and by tallying Correct Information Units (CIUs), a measure of the semantic content of participants' utterances (Nicholas & Brookshire, 1993). By identifying the specific aspects of spontaneous speech that are altered as a result of stimulation, we aimed to provide further insight into the specific linguistic processes improved by TMS.

METHOD

Participants

A total of 10 participants (3 female) ranging in age between 47 and 75 years (mean ± *SD*, 61.60 ± 8.32) took part. All participants had sustained a single left hemispheric unilateral ischaemic stroke (Figure 1) and were classified as having mild to moderate nonfluent aphasia by Boston Diagnostic Aphasia Examination tests (BDAE; Goodglass, Kaplan, & Barresi, 2001) administered at the initial screening. To be eligible for the study patients must have been able to produce meaningful words as well as phrases between 2–4 words in length during their baseline language evaluation. To ensure that participants were able to cooperate during testing they also must have had relatively intact language comprehension, operationally defined by performance at or above the 25th percentile on the BDAE subtests for word comprehension and commands. Additionally participants must have been able to name at least 3 items of the first 30 on the Boston Naming Test (Kaplan, Goodglass, & Weintraub, 2001) and an average of at least 3 pictures out of 20 when presented with 10 sets of picture naming stimuli taken from the Snodgrass and Vanderwart corpus (1980). All participants were at least 6 months post-stroke, had no other concurrent history of neurological or psychiatric disease or unstable medical conditions, and had no contra-indications to either MRI or TMS. The study was approved by the Institutional Review Board of the University of Pennsylvania, and all participants provided informed consent. Additional participant demographic, baseline performance, and lesion data are provided in Table 1.

STUDY OVERVIEW

At the start of the study all participants underwent baseline language assessment three times on average (range: 1–4). The baseline assessment included testing with

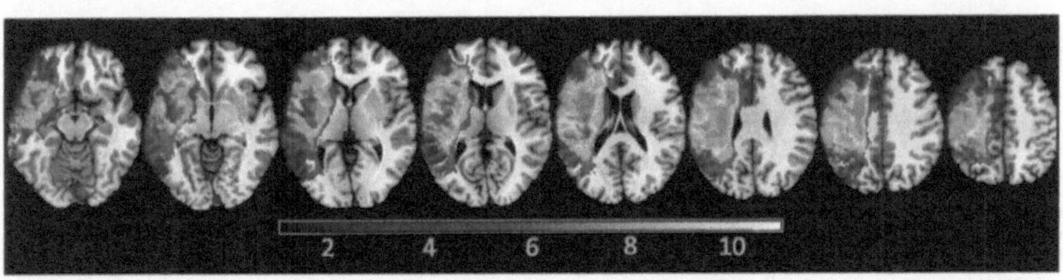

Figure 1. Lesion overlap for all 10 left MCA stroke participants mapped onto the Colin27 MNI template. The location of maximal overlap (bright orange) includes the left insula, Heschl's gyrus, and Rolandic operculum. To view this figure in colour, please see the online issue of the journal.

TABLE 1
Demographics, lesion descriptions, and aphasia severity measures for study participants

							Aphasia Severity		
Subject	*Sex*	*Age, y*	*Education, y*	*Time Since Stroke, mo*	*Lesion Distribution*	*Lesion Volume, cm³*	*Phrase length (BDAE), mean*	*Naming ability (BNT), (maximum 30)*	*Auditory Comprehension-Commands (BDAE), (maximum 15)*
					Real TMS				
1	M	60	18	87	Large MCA cortical and subcortical, including BA 44, 45, & 47	252.11	2.5	21	8
2	M	61	18	63	Large MCA cortical and subcortical, including BA 44, 45, & 47	130.91	2	7	14
3	M	51	14	45	Fronto-pariental cortical and subcortical, including interanal capsule, basal ganglia, BA 44, 45, & 47	134.03	3.5	27	15
4	F	71	18	48	Fronto-temporo-parietal subcortical greater than cortical, including internal capsule, basal ganglia & thalamus; M1 & IFG spared	91.65	5	20	11
5	M	60	24	6	Small fronto-temporo-parietal cortical and subcortical; minor involvement of corona radiata; IFG and insula spared	36.59	3	8	15
Mean (StdDev)		60.6 (±7.1)	18.4 (±3.6)	49.8 (±29.6)		129.1 (±79.2)	3.2 (±1.2)	16.6 (±8.7)	12.6 (±3.0)

(Continued)

TABLE 1
(Continued)

Subject	*Sex*	*Age, y*	*Education, y*	*Time Since Stroke, mo*	*Lesion Distribution*	*Lesion Volume, cm^3*	*Aphasia Severity*		
							Phrase length (BDAE), mean	*Naming ability (BNT), (maximum 30)*	*Auditory Comprehension-Commands (BDAE), (maximum 15)*
					Sham TMS				
1	M	65	12	29	Subcortical, including corona radiata, internal capsule, basal ganglia, & thalamus; IFG spared	53.02	2.5	13	11
2	F	65	16	20	Large MCA cortical & subcortical, including BA 44, 45, & 47	201.62	3	20	8
3	M	47	12	102	Cortical & subcortical, including internal capsule, basal ganglia, thalamus, M1, and BA 44; BA 45 & 47 spared	123.83	2.5	26	11
4	F	61	14	59	Large MCA cortical & subcortical, including BA 44, 45, & 47	178.99	1	17	14
5	M	75	18	83	Fronto-temporo-parietal subcortical, including corona radiata but sparing internal capsule and deep grey structures; IFG spared	118.49	3	21	11
	Mean (StdDev)	62.6 (±10.1)	14.4 (±2.6)	58.6 (±34.8)		135.2 (±58.1)	2.4 (±0.8)	19.4 (±4.8)	11.0 (±2.1)

the Cookie Theft Picture Description subtest of the BDAE, described further below. The average interval between initial and final baseline testing sessions was 33 days (SD = 34.16 days). Following baseline assessment each participant was randomised into one of two groups: One group (n = 5) received real rTMS while the other group (n = 5) initially received sham stimulation (sTMS). Statistically these two groups did not differ significantly with respect to age, lesion size, time since stroke onset, or initial measures of aphasia severity. There was a trend towards significance between the two groups with respect to years of education, $t(7.3) = 2.02$; $p = .081$, with a greater number of years of education in the rTMS group (18.4, SD = 3.6) than the sham group (14.4, SD = 2.6). Participants receiving real rTMS underwent a series of six sessions of rTMS applied to different sites in right IFG in order to identify the optimal target for stimulation. After an optimal site was identified for each individual participant, stimulation was administered to that site in 10 sessions over 12 days (daily sessions occurred Monday through Friday for 2 weeks with no stimulation on Saturday or Sunday), as described below. Participants subsequently completed a follow-up language assessment including Cookie Theft Picture Description 2 months following the completion of stimulation. Testing was not pursued immediately after discontinuation of stimulation because of concerns that repeating language tasks only a short interval after finishing baseline testing might elicit practice effects. Prior evidence (Hamilton et al., 2010) suggested that improvements in spontaneous speech due to rTMS could be observed after 2 months. Participants randomised to the sham group received sham rTMS during both the optimal target identification phase of the study as well as during the 10-session treatment phase. These participants completed a follow-up language assessment including the Cookie Theft Picture Description 2 months following sTMS, and subsequently crossed over into the real rTMS arm of the study, such that all participants in the study eventually received real rTMS. Study events are summarised in Figure 2.

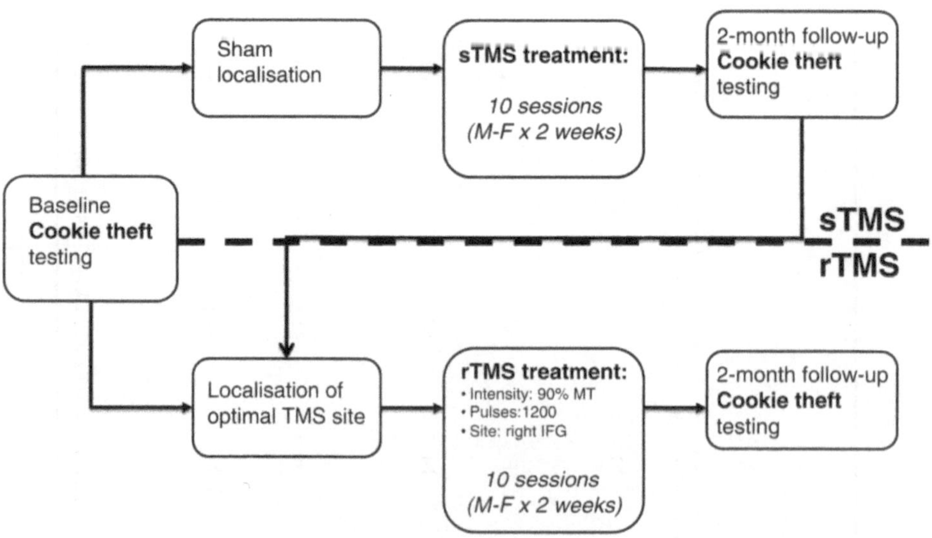

Figure 2. Outline of study events.

rTMS methods

Stimulation was administered with a Magstim Rapid transcranial magnetic stimulator, connected to a 70-mm diameter figure-of-eight coil (Magstim, Whitland, UK). A 3.0 Tesla Siemens Trio Scanner was used to collect high-resolution whole-brain T1-weighted images for each participant. The Brainsight system (Rogue Research, Montreal) was used to co-register MRI data with the location of the participant and coil in both phases of the study. The participant's resting motor threshold (RMT) was established according to published criteria (Rossini et al., 1994). Sham TMS was administered using the same setup, but with the coil perpendicular to the head so that only the rim of the coil contacted the head. During real stimulation the coil was oriented with the handle in a posterior and inferior direction approximately 45 degrees clockwise from the downward position. Real rTMS was delivered at an intensity of 90% RMT and a frequency of 1 Hz. During each of the 10 sessions of the treatment phase of the study participants in the real rTMS arm of the study received 1200 pulses of 1Hz rTMS at 90% RMT; participants in the sham arm 1200 pulses of sTMS.

Identification of optimal stimulation site

These methods are described in more detail elsewhere (Hamilton et al., 2010; Naeser et al., 2011). In six separate sessions conducted over 5 days (two sessions were conducted on the last day) different sites in the right inferior frontal lobe were stimulated with rTMS. During these sessions participants in the real rTMS arm of the study received 600 pulses of 1Hz rTMS at an intensity of 90% RMT, while participants in the sham arm received 600 pulses of sTMS. Sites included the region of the motor cortex corresponding to the mouth, a site on pars opercularis (BA 44), three separate sites on the pars triangularis (BA 45; designated in this study as the dorsal posterior, ventral posterior, and anterior pars triangularis), and the pars orbitalis (BA 47). Prior to and immediately following rTMS at each candidate site, participants performed a 40-item picture-naming task. As in previous work, responses that differed from the target by one phoneme were counted as correct (e.g., Naeser et al., 2005). As previously reported, a site was considered to be the optimal target for stimulation if a participant showed the greatest increase in naming accuracy after stimulation of that target and if the change in naming accuracy observed after stimulation of that target was greater than two times the standard deviation of the mean pre-stimulation performance across all sites (Hamilton et al., 2011). Consistent with prior investigations, for 9 out of 10 participants tested, the optimal site was in the right pars triangularis (RPTr); for one participant the optimal site was found to be in the right pars orbitalis (see Figure 3).

Stimulus presentation

Seated comfortably in a quiet testing environment, participants were presented with the "Cookie Theft" picture from the Boston Diagnostic Aphasia Examination by an examiner, and instructed to report everything they saw in the picture. Examiner interruptions were limited to general prompts (e.g., "what's happening here"); examiners did not point to or allude to specific content in the picture. There was no time limit for responses. Participants performed this task three times at baseline and after 2-month real rTMS follow-up. Participants randomised to the sham arm performed the task at

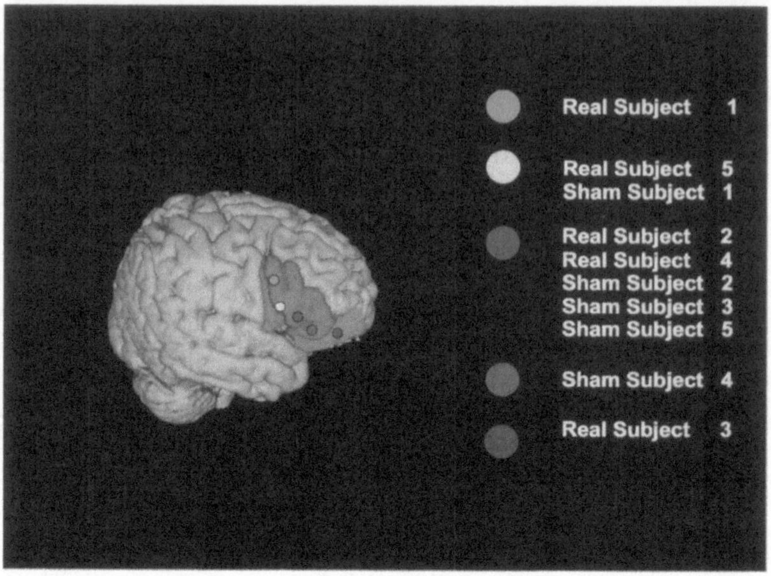

Figure 3. Right hemisphere overlay of optimal real TMS sites for the 10 participants in the study mapped onto the Colin27 MNI template. Participants are labelled as Real or Sham participants 1–5 (based on which type of treatment they received first, although the sites shown all correspond to their real TMS sites), and correspond with participant labels in Table 1. Shading indicates gyral anatomy: Green = pars opercularis, Red = pars triangularis, Yellow = pars orbitalis. To view this figure in colour, please see the online issue of the journal.

2-month sTMS follow-up as well. Speech samples were recorded digitally and coded offline by an experimenter (CN). The order of sessions was randomised during coding and the coder was blinded with respect to participant condition and session order.

Measures of fluency

A variety of elements were quantified in each speech sample using QPA (Saffran et al., 1989). We categorised these variables based on four aspects of speech fluency: discourse productivity, sentence productivity, grammatical accuracy, and lexical selection (Gordon, 2006).

Discourse productivity. This category described the production of words related to the picture stimulus. Narrative words (NW) were defined as the total words minus stereotyped utterances, task-related comments, or comments cued by the narrator. The number of narrative words that were verbs and nouns was recorded, as was the number of unique verbs and nouns. Closed-class words (CCW) were defined as the number of narrative words that were determiners, pronouns, conjunctions, and prepositions; other words were counted as open-class words (OCW). The duration and rate (measured in words per minute) of participants' speech samples were also recorded.

Sentence productivity. This category quantified the length and complexity of sentences. Mean sentence length was defined as the average of the number of words per utterance containing a noun and a main verb. Median utterance length referred to the number of narrative words per utterance. The sentence elaboration index is a composite score of the number of narrative words per phrase for both noun and verb phrases. The embedding index is the proportion of sentences that contain an embedded clause.

Grammatical accuracy. This category included the proportion of sentences that were well-formed, in that they contain a subject, predicate, and direct object (where necessary). The auxiliary score was defined as an index of the morphological complexity of the main verb of the sentence. The inflexion index is a measure of verbs that have been changed from their base form.

Lexical selection. This category measured the usage words relative to other words in an utterance. The proportion of CCWs reflected the number of CCWs relative to the total number of narrative words. Similarly, the proportion of pronouns and the proportion of verbs relative to total narrative words were also measured.

In addition to QPA, speech samples were also scored with respect to Correct Information Units (CIUs), which were defined as the number of words that were intelligible, accurate, informative, and relevant to the eliciting stimulus (see Nicholas & Brookshire, 1993).

Analysis

We pursued a within-participants comparison contrasting performance 2 months after real rTMS to baseline performance in all participants ($N = 10$), using raw performance scores as dependent variables. Because we had strong a priori predictions about the direction of change likely to be induced by rTMS based on prior evidence (e.g., Barwood et al., 2011; Hamilton et al., 2010; Naeser et al., 2005), one-tailed t-tests were employed. We also used within-participants comparisons to contrast 2-month follow-up performance to baseline performance after sTMS in the subset of participants receiving sham stimulation ($N = 5$), using raw performance scores as dependent variables. To confirm that significant rTMS vs baseline effects did not result from practice effects or bias due to unblinding in patients crossed over from the sham arm to the real rTMS arm, we performed a between-participants comparison contrasting the proportion change from baseline to 2-month follow-up on each study measure in patients who received sTMS ($N = 5$) to those who received rTMS initially ($N = 5$), using independent samples one-tailed t-tests. For all independent samples t-tests (using PASW 18), we used a Levene's test for equality of variances to test for homogeneity of variance. When assumptions of homogeneity of variance were not met, we adjusted the degrees of freedom using the Welch-Satterthwaite method. We did not make any explicit corrections for multiple comparisons as many of the variables were complementary, consisting of subdivisions of other variables (e.g., total nouns and verbs as part of narrative words). Furthermore, it has been suggested that, in exploratory studies, one should not correct for multiple comparisons but instead present the p-values for all tests for interpretation (see Rothman, 1990). Note that, given the number of comparisons we are presenting in the paper (21), we would expect about one comparison to be significant if the data were generated at chance.

RESULTS

Comparison of real rTMS to baseline

All participants tolerated stimulation without complaint of physical discomfort or other adverse effects. First we used *t*-tests to observe if there were any differences in baseline performance between participants who received real rTMS initially versus those who received real rTMS after sTMS. For all 21 dependent variables we did not find any significant differences between the two groups in baseline performance (average *p*-value, .521, range, .131–.979), performance at 2-month follow-up (average *p*-value, .494; range, .059–.984), or proportional change from baseline (average *p*-value, .468; range, .113–.879). Therefore results from these two groups were collapsed for the first analysis. The participants demonstrated a significant increase in discourse productivity (see Figure 4), as shown by the significant increase in the number of narrative words 2 months post-treatment compared to baseline, $t(9) = -2.07$, $p = .035$. Within narrative words, we found that participants demonstrated a significant increase in production of open-class words, $t(9) = -2.02$, $p = .037$, closed-class words, $t(9) = -1.95$, $p = .042$, total number of verbs, $t(9) = -2.28$, $p = .024$, unique nouns, $t(9) = -2.02$, $p = .037$, and marginal effects for total number of nouns, $t(9) = -1.82$, $p = .051$, and unique words, $t(9) = -1.63$, $p = .068$. We found no effect for unique verbs, $t(9) = -0.015$, $p = .494$. Consistent with the notion that participants were generating more words relevant to the picture stimulus, there was a trend towards an increase in the number of CIUs generated, $t(9) = -1.60$, $p = .072$. These increases in narrative productivity were not due to participants speaking for longer

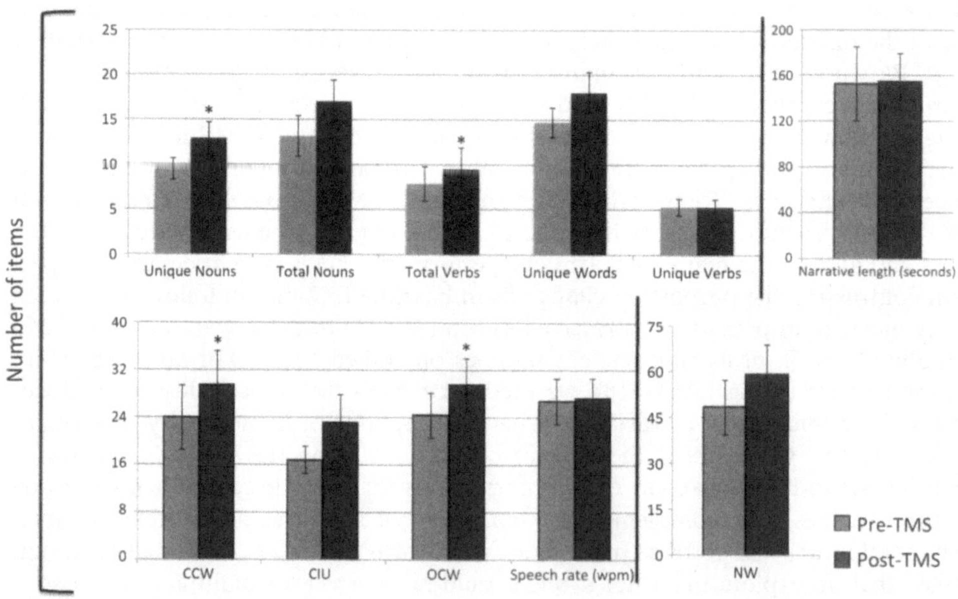

Figure 4. Performance on measures of discourse productivity before and 2 months after receiving real rTMS ($N = 10$). Vertical lines represent standard error. Significant improvement ($p = <.05$) is indicated by "*". NW = Narrative Words; CCW = Closed-class Words; OCW = Open-class Words; CIU = Correct Information Units.

periods of time, as there was only a 1.6-second difference in mean passage length, $t(9) = -0.13$, $p = .449$, between baseline and 2-month follow-up. Nor were participants simply speaking more rapidly, since there was no significant change in speech rate $t(8) = -2.70$, $p = .397$. However, participants showed a marginally significant increase in the total number of utterances before versus after treatment, $t(9) = -1.68$, $p = .064$, and also trend toward significance, $t(9) = -1.72$, $p = .059$, in the percentage of narrative words over total words uttered 2 months after treatment (73.6%) versus at baseline (69.5%).

There was no significant improvement among participants receiving sTMS for any measure of discourse productivity. In contrast to findings within the category of discourse productivity, no significant changes in performance were seen along any variables in the other three fluency categories—sentence productivity, grammatical accuracy, and lexical selection—for either the real rTMS or sTMS conditions (see Figure 5 a–c; see also Supplementary Table 1).

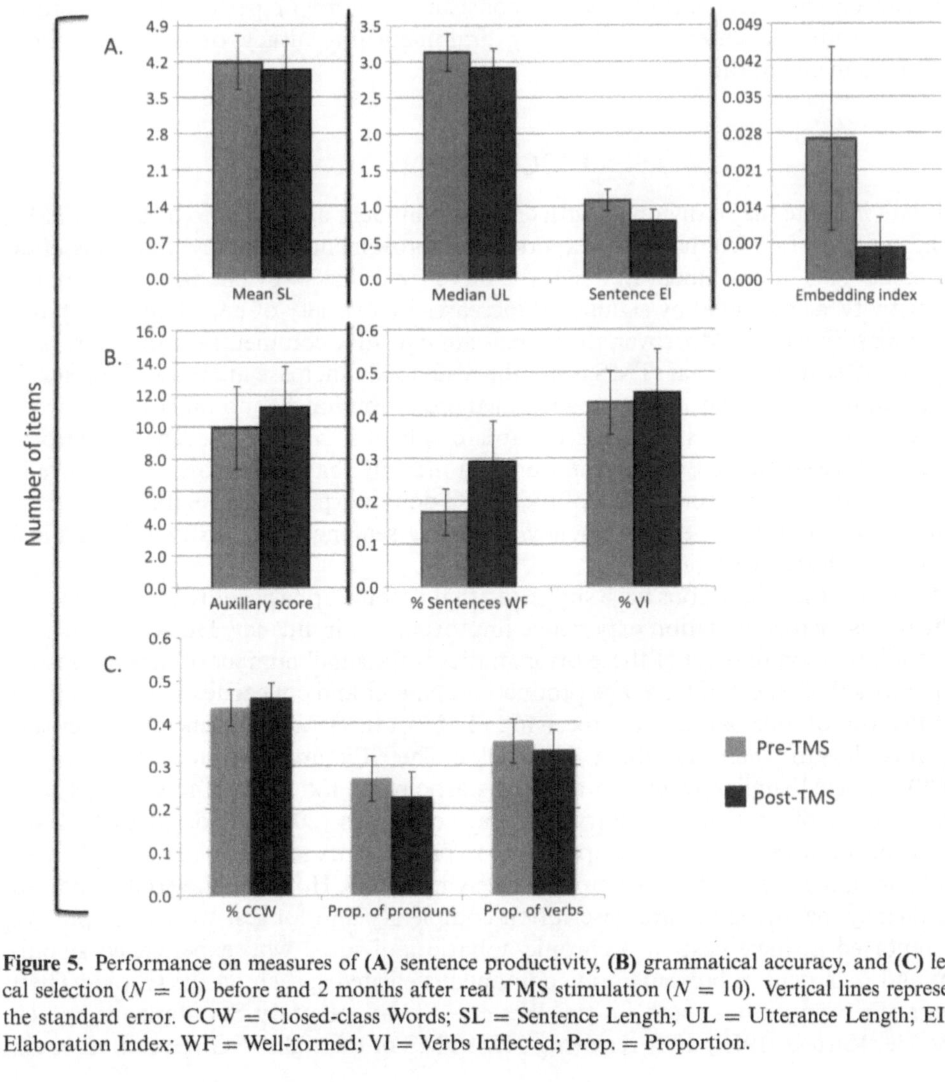

Figure 5. Performance on measures of **(A)** sentence productivity, **(B)** grammatical accuracy, and **(C)** lexical selection ($N = 10$) before and 2 months after real TMS stimulation ($N = 10$). Vertical lines represent the standard error. CCW = Closed-class Words; SL = Sentence Length; UL = Utterance Length; EI = Elaboration Index; WF = Well-formed; VI = Verbs Inflected; Prop. = Proportion.

Comparison of real rTMS to sTMS

Unfortunately the statistical power to make comparisons between participants who had initially received rTMS compared to those who had initially received sTMS was limited due to the small sample size. There was a significantly greater increase from baseline in the use of closed-class words for participants receiving rTMS compared to participants receiving sTMS, $t(7.4) = -2.10$, $p = .036$. There were also trends towards greater change from baseline in participants receiving rTMS compared to participants receiving sTMS for other measures of discourse productivity, including narrative words, $t(6.77) = -1.87$, $p = .053$, unique words, $t(7.73) = -1.65$, $p = .070$, unique nouns, $t(6.32) = -1.48$, $p = .094$, unique verbs, $t(7.47) = -1.78$, $p = .058$, open-class words, $t(7.54) = -1.59$, $p = .076$, and CIUs, $t(5.3) = 1.7$, $p = .072$. No significant differences or trends were found for any measures of sentence productivity, grammatical accuracy, or lexical selection (all p-values $> .1$). Finally there was a very consistent direction of numerical change across all measures of narrative word generation, with participants receiving rTMS showing a greater improvement from baseline than participants receiving sTMS. No consistent pattern of performance emerged across measures of sentence productivity, grammatical accuracy, or lexical selection (see Supplementary Table 2).

DISCUSSION

Our data indicate that individuals with chronic nonfluent aphasia who undergo rTMS of the right inferior frontal gyrus experience improvement in fluency 2 months after treatment. This improvement in fluency is driven specifically by changes in discourse productivity, as indicated by significant increases in a variety of narrative word types following stimulation. Moreover, the increase in narrative comments exhibited by participants after receiving real rTMS is not the result of an increase in the speaking speed or duration, but instead reflects a shift in the distribution of utterances away from irrelevant non-narrative statements towards comments that are relevant to the presented picture stimulus. By contrast, our data indicate that participants with chronic nonfluent aphasia receiving rTMS of the RIFG do not experience a significant benefit with respect to other aspects of fluency, including sentence complexity, grammatical accuracy, or lexical selection.

A few prior investigations have suggested that chronic aphasic individuals receiving right hemisphere stimulation experience improvements in fluency. However, one significant limitation of most of these prior studies is the small number of measures used to quantify this aspect of language production. Naeser and colleagues (2005) reported that two out of four participants receiving rTMS of the IFG experienced an increase in phrase length when describing the Cookie Theft Picture. Martin and colleagues (2009) reported similar results in a single participant. Extending these results to a larger cohort of participants, Barwood and colleagues (2011) reported that rTMS treatment improved picture description in six participants receiving real rTMS treatment compared to six other participants receiving sTMS. However, they only reported two fluency measures: picture description complexity and longest words per phrase. We reported a single case of a chronic aphasic individual who experienced significant and persistent improvement in spontaneous elicited speech on the Cookie Theft Picture Description task and on the Western Aphasia Battery Spontaneous speech subscale (Kertesz, 1982) after receiving 1Hz rTMS of the right IFG (Hamilton et al.,

2010). Unlike prior studies we examined a variety of speech production indices, and found that the participant experienced significant increases in narrative words, different nouns, mean sentence length, and closed-class words per sentence. We also recently reported a single case in which a chronically aphasic participant experienced an increase in the number of unique words employed and a marginal increase in the CIUs during a picture description 2 months after receiving real rTMS (Turkeltaub, Coslett, et al., 2011). The current study builds on our prior findings, confirming in one of the largest reported cohorts of chronic aphasic participants receiving rTMS to date that inhibitory rTMS of the RIFG improves fluency, and clarifying that this effect is related specifically to improved discourse productivity.

The mechanisms by which rTMS of the RIFG improves discourse productivity in individuals with chronic nonfluent aphasia are unclear. However, the performance patterns observed in our participants militate against certain explanations. One possible account for the increase in narrative words is that TMS facilitates speech via mechanisms that are only indirectly related to language functions, for example by diminishing frontal lobe mediated behavioural inhibition or by modulating arousal. However, this account would predict that participants would experience an overall increase in speech production, and does not adequately explain why our participants experience a shift in the distribution of their words towards narrative utterances and away from non-narrative utterances. Neither do our results accord with the notion that rTMS is principally affecting motor aspects of speech production, since this also would not explain a shift towards narrative utterances.

While our findings help to identify which aspects of language production are affected by RIFG rTMS, they do not resolve ongoing debate regarding the neural mechanisms mediating stimulation effects in persons with chronic aphasia. Much of this debate centres on the role of right hemisphere structures in aphasia recovery. One account is that the right hemisphere is deleterious to language recovery, possibly due to the presence of inhibitory interhemispheric connections from the right to the left hemisphere that diminish the recovery of perilesional left hemisphere language areas. A competing account argues that the role of the right hemisphere in aphasia recovery is largely compensatory, and that inhibitory rTMS of specific right hemisphere sites modulates the efficiency of compensatory right hemisphere networks (Hamilton et al., 2011). Based on data from prior imaging studies (Turkeltaub, Messing, Norise, & Hamilton, 2011) and from one specific participant with chronic aphasia who received rTMS and then experienced a second stroke affecting her right hemisphere (Turkeltaub, Coslett, et al., 2011), we have argued that the role of some right hemisphere regions appears to be compensatory while that of other regions appears to interfere with language processing (Hamilton et al., 2011).

One plausible explanation for the current results is that rTMS of the RIFG selectively improves lexical-semantic access. Lexical-semantic access is often profoundly delayed in participants with non-fluent aphasia (Edwards, 1995). Participants who have received inhibitory stimulation may be better able to retrieve the appropriate representations of words and word meanings, and are thus better able to generate more narrative utterances that are relevant to the picture stimulus presented to them. Supporting this notion, all of the study measures in which our participants showed improvement involved accessing words in various categories, with no improvement in measures of grammatical complexity or sentence construction. Improvement in lexical-semantic processing is also consistent with the already established finding that stimulation of this region improves naming, a process that also relies in large part on the retrieval of accurate lexical-semantic representations (Martin et al., 2004; Naeser et al., 2005, 2010; Winhuisen et al., 2005). The fact that the optimal site during TMS site-finding in our study is the RPTr in 9 out of 10 participants further suggests that inhibition of this specific site has a facilitative effect on lexical-semantic selection (see also Naeser et al., 2011). Furthermore, it has also been shown that rTMS presented to the RPTr in patients with chronic nonfluent aphasia induces changes in the N400 signal (Barwood et al., 2011), an ERP marker that has been associated with lexical-semantic aspects of language processing (Brown & Hagoort, 1993; Halgren et al., 2002; Kutas & Federmeier, 2000; Simos, Basile, & Papanicolaou, 1997).

The notion that TMS of the right PTr might selectively affect lexical-semantic processing is consistent with converging evidence suggesting that individuals with aphasia engage right hemisphere structures during language processing and that these right hemisphere areas are functionally specific. A recent meta-analysis of neuroimaging studies in aphasia indicates that many right hemisphere perisylvian regions that are activated during language tasks in aphasic individuals are homotopic and functionally homologous with left hemisphere areas that normally subserve language in normal persons (Turkeltaub, Messing, et al., 2011). By contrast the right PTr, while homotopic in location with an area of activation in controls, was not homologous with respect to functional activity. Turkeltaub and colleagues suggested that activation observed in the right PTr in aphasic individuals may be dysfunctional, a view further supported by studies that have associated increased right IFG activation with overt naming errors in aphasic participants (Postman-Caucheteux et al., 2010). A number of studies have demonstrated that, in healthy participants, more ventral-anterior regions of the left IFG (including PTr) are preferentially involved in lexical-semantic processing, while posterior-dorsal areas (including the pars opercularis; POp) are preferentially involved in phonology (Bookheimer, 2002; Gough, Nobre, & Devlin, 2005; Hagoort, 2005; Poldrack et al., 1999). Moreover, Hartwigsen and colleagues (2010) found that in healthy individuals disruption of the right POp with TMS resulted in worsened performance on a phonological selection task, while disruption of the right PTr had no effect on a matched semantic task. This finding suggests that, although it is homotopic with a LIFG region that mediates lexical-semantic processing in normal persons, the right PTr is poorly suited to support recovery of lexical-semantic processing after LIFG injury. This is consistent with functional imaging data in aphasia demonstrating that left hemisphere activation was associated with phonemic naming errors, but right hemisphere activity was associated with semantic naming errors (Fridriksson, Baker, & Moser, 2009). By this account, inhibition of overactivity in the right PTr might result in suppression of an inefficient node in the remodelled language network that otherwise contributes deleteriously to lexical-semantic processing.

The current study has limitations. Even though this is one of the largest studies to report on the effects of rTMS on language ability in persons with chronic nonfluent aphasia the study is still underpowered, and additional investigations in larger cohorts of participants are needed to establish the impact of rTMS on measures of fluency more definitively. Also the number of speech samples gathered from each participant was relatively low compared to the volume of data collected in the original studies validating the QPA (Berndt, Wayland, Rochon, Saffran, & Schwarz, 2000) and the use of CIUs (Nicholas & Brookshire, 1993). Baseline testing was not repeated for participants who initially received sham stimulation prior to receiving real rTMS. While it is therefore possible that introduction of sham rTMS and a 2-month time interval could have resulted in a different baseline level of performance for these individuals, the absence of change on any study measure between baseline and 2-month follow-up in participants who had received sTMS argues against this claim. Finally, owing to the difference in sensory experience between real and sham stimulation, we cannot exclude the possibility that some participants were not fully blinded to their condition when receiving sTMS. It should be noted, however, that no participant had received TMS prior to the study and therefore would not have had expectations regarding the sensory experiences associated with TMS. Despite these caveats, the current data suggest that in addition to improving naming ability rTMS may be a promising technique for remediating dysfluency, one of the most debilitating deficits for many patients with chronic aphasia.

REFERENCES

Barwood, C. H., Murdoch, B. E., Whelan, B. M., Lloyd, D., Riek, S., O'Sullivan, J. D., . . . Wong, A. (2011). Improved language performance subsequent to low-frequency rTMS in patients with chronic non-fluent aphasia post-stroke. *European Journal of Neurology*, *18*, 935–943.

Berndt, R. S., Wayland, S., Rochon, E., Saffran, E., & Schwartz, M. (2000). *Quantitative production analysis: A training manual for the analysis of aphasic sentence production*. Philadelphia, PA: Psychology Press.

Bookheimer, S. (2002). Functional MRI of language: New approaches to understanding the cortical organization of semantic processing. *Annual Review of Neuroscience*, *25*, 151–88.

Brown, C., & Hargoort, P. (1993). The processing nature of the N400: Evidence from masked priming. *Journal of Cognitive Neuroscience*, *5*, 34–44.

Edwards, S. (1995). Profiling fluent aphasic spontaneous speech: A comparison of two methodologies. *European Journal of Disorders of Communication*, *30*, 333–345.

Fridriksson, J., Baker, J. M., & Moser, D. (2009). Cortical mapping of naming errors in aphasia. *Human Brain Mapping*, *30*, 2487–2498.

Gleason, J. B., Goodglass, H., Green, E., Ackerman, N., & Hyde, M. R. (1975). The retrieval of syntax in Broca's aphasia. *Brain & Language*, *2*, 451–471.

Goodglass, H., Kaplan, E., & Barresi, B. (2001). *Boston Diagnostic Aphasia Examination (BDAE)*. Philadelphia, PA: Lippincott, Williams & Wilkins.

Gordon, J. K. (2006). A quantitative production analysis of picture description. *Aphasiology*, *20*, 188–204.

Gough, P. M., Nobre, A. C., & Devlin, J. T. (2005). Dissociating linguistic processes in the left inferior frontal cortex with transcranial magnetic stimulation. *Journal of Neuroscience*, *25*, 8010–8016.

Hagoort, P. (2005). On Broca, brain, and binding: A new framework. *Trends in Cognitive Science*, *9*, 416–423.

Halgren, E., Dhond, R. P., Christensen, N., Van Petten, C., Marinkovic, K., Lewine, J. D., & Dale, A. M. (2002). N400-like magnetoencephalography responses modulated by semantic context, word frequency, and lexical class in sentences. *Neuroimage*, *17*, 1101–1116.

Hamilton, R. H., Chrysikou, E. G., & Coslett, B. (2011). Mechanisms of aphasia recovery after stroke and the role of noninvasive brain stimulation. *Brain & Language*, *118*, 40–50.

Hamilton, R. H., Sanders, L., Benson, J., Faseyitan, O., Norise, C., Naeser, M., . . . Coslett, H. B. (2010). Stimulating conversation: Enhancement of elicited propositional speech in a patient with chronic non-fluent aphasia following transcranial magnetic stimulation. *Brain & Language*, *113*, 45–50.

Hartwigsen, G., Price, C. J., Baumgaertner, A., Geiss, G., Koehnke, M., Ulmer, S., & Siebner, H. R. (2010). The right posterior inferior frontal gyrus contributes to phonological word decisions in the healthy brain: Evidence from dual-site TMS. *Neuropsychologia*, *48*, 3155–3163.

Kaplan, E., Goodglass, H., & Weintraub, S. (2001). *Boston Naming Test (BNT)*. Austin, TX: Lippincott Williams & Wilkins.

Kertesz, A. (1982). *Western aphasia battery*. New York, NY: Grune & Stratton.

Kolk, H., & Heeschen, C. (1990). Adaptation symptoms and impairment symptoms in Broca's aphasia. *Aphasiology*, *4*, 221–231.

Kutas, M., & Federmeier, K. D. (2000). Electrophysiology reveals semantic memory use in language comprehension. *Trends in Cognitive Science*, *4*, 463–470.

Martin, P. I., Naeser, M. A., Ho, M., Doron, K. W., Kurland, J., Kaplan, J., . . . Pascual-Leone, A. (2009). Overt naming fMRI pre- and post-TMS: Two nonfluent aphasia patients, with and without improved naming post-TMS. *Brain & Language*, *111*, 20–35.

Martin, P. I., Naeser, M. A., Theoret, H., Tormos, J. M., Nicholas, M., Kurland, J., . . . Pascual-Leone, A. (2004). Transcranial magnetic stimulation as a complementary treatment for aphasia. *Seminars in Speech and Language*, *25*, 181–191.

Naeser, M. A., Martin, P. I., Nicholas, M., Baker, E. H., Seekins, H., Kobayashi, M., . . . Pascual-Leone, A. (2005). Improved picture naming in chronic aphasia after TMS to part of right Broca's area: An open-protocol study. *Brain & Language*, *93*, 95–105.

Naeser, M. A., Martin, P. I., Theoret, H., Kobayashi, M., Fregni, F., Nicholas, M., . . . Pascual-Leone, A. (2011). TMS suppression of right pars triangularis, but not pars opercularis, improves naming in aphasia. *Brain & Language*, *119*, 206–213.

Naeser, M. A., Martin, P. I., Treglia, E., Ho, M., Kaplan, E., Bashir, S., . . . Pascual-Leone, A. (2010). Research with rTMS in the treatment of aphasia. *Restorative Neurology and Neuroscience*, *28*, 511–529.

Nicholas, L. E., & Brookshire, R. H. (1993). A system for quantifying the informativeness and efficiency of the connected speech of adults with aphasia. *Journal of Speech and Hearing Research*, *36*, 338–350.

Poldrack, R. A., Wagner, A. D., Prull, M. W., Desmond, J. E., Glover, G. H., & Gabrieli, J. D. (1999). Functional specialization for semantic and phonological processing in the left inferior prefrontal cortex. *Neuroimage*, *10*, 15–35.

Postman-Caucheteux, W. A., Birn, R. M., Pursley, R. H., Butman, J. A., Solomon, J. M., Picchioni, D., . . . Braun, A. R. (2010). Single-trial fMRI shows contralesional activity linked to overt naming errors in chronic aphasic patients. *Journal of Cognitive Neuroscience*, *22*, 1299–1318.

Rochon, E., Saffran, E. M., Berndt, R. S., & Schwartz, M. F. (2000). Quantitative analysis of aphasic sentence production: Further development and new data. *Brain & Language*, *72*, 193–218.

Rossini, P. M., Barker, A. T., Berardelli, A., Caramia, M. D., Caruso, G., Cracco, R. Q., . . . Tomberg, C. (1994). Non-invasive electrical and magnetic stimulation of the brain, spinal cord and roots: Basic principles and procedures for routine clinical application. Report of an IFCN Committee. *Electroencephalography and Clinical Neurophysiology*, *91*, 79–92.

Rothman, K. J. (1990). No adjustments are needed for multiple comparisons. *Epidemiology*, *1*, 43–46.

Saffran, E. M., Berndt, R. S., & Schwartz, M. F. (1989). The quantitative analysis of agrammatic production: Procedure and data. *Brain & Language*, *37*, 440–479.

Simos, P. G., Basile, L. F., & Papanicolaou, A. C. (1997). Source localization of the N400 response in a sentence-reading paradigm using evoked magnetic fields and magnetic resonance imaging. *Brain Research*, *762*, 29–39.

Snodgrass, J. G., & Vanderwart, M. (1980). A standardized set of 260 pictures: Norms for name agreement, image agreement, familiarity, and visual complexity. *Journal of Experimental Psychology: Human Learning*, *6*, 174–215.

Turkeltaub, P. E., Coslett, H. B., Thomas, A. L., Faseyitan, O., Benson, J., Norise, C., & Hamilton, R. H. (2011). The right hemisphere is not unitary in its role in aphasia recovery. *Cortex*. Advance online publication.

Turkeltaub, P. E., Messing, S., Norise, C., & Hamilton, R. H. (2011). Are networks for residual language function and recovery consistent across aphasic patients? *Neurology*, *76*, 1726–1734.

Weiduschat, N., Thiel, A., Rubi-Fessen, I., Hartmann, A., Kessler, J., Merl, P., . . . Heiss, W. D. (2011). Effects of repetitive transcranial magnetic stimulation in aphasic stroke: A randomised controlled pilot study. *Stroke*, *42*, 409–415.

Winhuisen, L., Thiel, A., Schumacher, B., Kessler, J., Rudolf, J., Haupt, W. F., & Heiss, W. D. (2005). Role of the contralateral inferior frontal gyrus in recovery of language function in poststroke aphasia: A combined repetitive transcranial magnetic stimulation and positron emission tomography study. *Stroke*, *36*, 1759–1763.

APHASIOLOGY, 2012, 26 (9), 1169–1191

Can tDCS enhance treatment of aphasia after stroke?

Rachel Holland and Jenny Crinion

Institute of Cognitive Neuroscience, University College London, London, UK

Background: Recent advances in the application of transcranial direct current stimulation (tDCS) in healthy populations have led to the exploration of the technique as an adjuvant method to traditional speech therapies in patients with post-stroke aphasia.
Aims: The purpose of the review is: (i) to review the features of tDCS that make it an attractive tool for research and potential future use in clinical contexts; (ii) to describe recent studies exploring the facilitation of language performance using tDCS in post-stroke aphasia; (iii) to explore methodological considerations of tDCS that may be key to understanding tDCS in treatment of aphasia post stroke; and (iv) to highlight several caveats and outstanding questions that need to be addressed in future work.
Main Contribution: This review aims to highlight our current understanding of the methodological and theoretical issues surrounding the use of tDCS as an adjuvant tool in the treatment of language difficulties after stroke.
Conclusions: Preliminary evidence shows that tDCS may be a useful tool to complement treatment of aphasia, particularly for speech production in chronic stroke patients. To build on this exciting work, further systematic research is needed to understand the mechanisms of tDCS-induced effects, its application to current models of aphasia recovery, and the complex interactions between different stimulation parameters and language rehabilitation techniques. The potential of tDCS is to optimise language rehabilitation techniques and promote long-term recovery of language. A stimulating future for aphasia rehabilitation!

Keywords: Transcranial direct current stimulation; Post stroke aphasia; Recovery.

Language-based therapeutic interventions for post-stoke aphasia are effective at alleviating some degree of language impairment (Kendall et al., 2008; Nickels, 2002; Vitali et al., 2007). The dose of speech and language therapy (SLT) delivered may have a critical effect on recovery (Breitenstein et al., 2009; Brindley, Copeland, Demain, & Martyn, 1989; Meinzer, Djunja, Barthel, Elbert, & Rockstroh, 2005; Meinzer et al., 2004; Poeck, Huber, & Willmes, 1989). The idea being that for beneficial therapeutic outcome "more is better". Indeed, in studies that report positive therapy outcomes patients were provided with, on average, a total of 98.4 hours of therapy, while studies in which no improvement was observed, only 43.6 hours of therapy was delivered (Bhogal, Teasell, Foley, & Speechley, 2003). Although modest evidence exists for the efficacy of more intensive treatment and constraint induced language therapy (CILT) in individuals with chronic stroke-induced aphasia (Barthel, Meinzer, Djundja, &

Address correspondence to: Rachel Holland, Institute of Cognitive Neuroscience, University College London, 17 Queen Square, London WC1N 3AR, UK. E-mail: rachel.holland@ucl.ac.uk

http://dx.doi.org/10.1080/02687038.2011.616925

Rockstroh, 2008; Cherney, Patterson, Raymer, Frymark, & Schooling, 2008; Meinzer et al., 2004, 2005; Pulvermuller et al., 2001), extensive language therapy, whether delivered intensively or not, is difficult to administer with limited clinical resources not least because significantly more people withdraw from intensive SLT than conventional SLT (Kelly, Brady, & Enderby, 2010). Consequently one approach may be to consider adjuncts to therapy that may facilitate treatment, such as brain stimulation interventions. The facilitation of performance could manifest in (i) an increase to the total amount of learning achieved, such that a higher performance level is reached, or (ii) an increased rate at which learning is achieved, such that the same maximum performance is ultimately achieved as with standard therapy alone but over a different timescale, i.e., with less hours of behavioural therapy. It is not clear what form of stimulation, for example repetitive transcranial magnetic stimulation (TMS), transcranial direct current stimulation (tDCS), or epidural electrical stimulation (EES) is most effective and clinically appropriate. However, tDCS is easier and less expensive, and theoretically could be even self-administered, while TMS requires special equipment and trained health professionals, and it carries a seizure risk; EES, on the other hand, is an invasive method that effectively limits the range of its application. In this paper we summarise results from tDCS studies that aim to elicit improvements in language performance and language learning in chronic post-stroke aphasic patients.

The translation of tDCS studies of language from healthy participants into aphasic patients has been limited. To date only four studies have reported data from post-stroke aphasic speakers (see Table 1). Although the number of studies is small, there is preliminary and exciting evidence that tDCS may play a role in aphasia rehabilitation. However, before we start our review of these studies, in Section 1 we briefly recap some of the basic mechanisms of tDCS that are relevant to the treatment of post-stroke aphasic patients. For a more comprehensive work detailing the mechanism of tDCS, TMS, and an overview of both methods we direct readers to excellent papers by Nitsche et al. (2008), Jahanshahi and Rothwell (2000), and Miniussi et al. (2008) respectively. For a review of the normative literature using tDCS to modulate language performance see Floël (2012). In Section 2 we review recent evidence for a facilitatory role of tDCS on naming performance in post-stroke aphasic patients, and in Section 3 we discuss several methodological parameters that, at present, remain unclear and require further consideration if tDCS is to be developed as a realistic therapeutic tool. We conclude in Section 4 by highlighting a number of caveats and questions that need to be addressed before tDCS may be clinically useful in aphasia rehabilitation. It is hoped that, by doing so, new insights and novel research approaches into the complex nature of aphasia and its treatment might lead to advances in the improvement of therapy outcomes in chronic post-stroke aphasic patients.

METHOD OF tDCS AND CONSIDERATIONS IN A DAMAGED BRAIN

In recent decades, tDCS has been re-evaluated and shown to reliably modulate human cortical function by inducing prolonged yet reversible shifts of cortical excitability. As such, it has been re-introduced as a non-invasive tool to guide neuroplasticity and modulate cortical function. tDCS relies on tonic stimulation of the cortex via the application of a direct, constant current flow of low intensity (1–2 mA) between two electrodes applied to the scalp over a relatively extended period of time (e.g., 5–20 minutes). This technique has been shown to elicit polarity-dependent changes

TABLE 1
tDCS and language performance in post-stroke aphasia

Authors	*n*	*Lesion location*	*Time post stroke in months (range)*	*Design*	*Stimulation*	*Stimulation parameters*	*Intervention*	*Exposure*	*Task*	*Results*	*Overall Mean % age change*	*Duration of effect*
Monti et al. (2008)	8	3 – L frontal 3 – L fronto-parietal 2 – L fronto-temporoparietal	47.2 (24–96)	Crossover Sham controlled 1 wk between sessions	A, C, S	2mA 10 min Left fronto-temporal cortex	Offline	Single	Picture naming	Accuracy significantly improved after cathodal, not anodal stimulation No effects in reaction time	10.6%	No follow-up data reported
Baker et al. (2010)	10	3 – L frontal 4 – L temporoparietal 1 – L fronto-parietal 1 – L fronto-temporoparietal 1 – L temporal	64.6 (10–42)	Crossover Randomised Sham controlled 1 wk between sessions	A, S	1mA 20 min Left frontal-precentral	Online	5 days	Spoken WPM	Accuracy significantly improved for treated items after anodal stimulation compared to sham	8.4%	1 week post-treatment

(*Continued*)

TABLE 1
(Continued)

Authors	n	Lesion location	Time post stroke in months (range)	Design	Stimulation	Stimulation parameters	Intervention	Exposure	Task	Results	Overall Mean % age change	Duration of effect
Fiori et al. (2010)	3	2 – L frontal (1 subcortical only) 1 – L fronto-temporoparietal	44 (21–71)	Crossover Randomised Sham controlled 1 wk between sessions	A, S	1mA 20 min Left Wernicke's area (CP5)	Online	5 days	Picture naming	Accuracy significantly improved on day 5 compared to day 1 after anodal stimulation	20.5%	3 weeks post-treatment (2 patients tested only)
Fridriksson et al. (2011)	8	All had posterior cortical or subcortical lesions	58.4 (10–150)	Crossover Randomised Sham controlled 3 wks between sessions	A, S	1mA 20 min Left posterior cortex	Online	5 days	Spoken WPM	Reaction time significantly faster after anodal compared to sham stimulation in 7/8 patients	38.2%	3 weeks post-treatment

A = anodal stimulation, C = cathodal stimulation, S = sham stimulation, WPM = word-picture match.

in cortical excitability depending on the orientation of the stimulation electrodes (Nitsche & Paulus, 2000). In the motor cortex, anodal stimulation increases neuronal excitability whereas cathodal stimulation reduces excitability (Antal, Nitsche, Kruse, et al., 2004b; Kincses, Antal, Nitsche, Bartfai, & Paulus, 2004). Furthermore, emerging evidence suggests that the effects of tDCS can persist beyond the period of stimulation (Nitsche & Paulus, 2001; Nitsche, Schauenburg, et al., 2003), with changes in task performance reported as late as 6–12 months post-intervention (Cohen Kadosh, Soskic, Iuculano, Kanai, & Walsh, 2010; Dockery, Hueckel-Weng, Birbaumer, & Plewnia, 2009; Reis et al., 2009).

Although both TMS and tDCS are forms of non-invasive brain stimulation, it should be kept in mind that the effects of TMS and tDCS cannot be assumed to be the same and further research is needed to determine the mechanisms underlying the effects of each technique on the brain. The effects of stimulation on language function, its cortical network, and its behavioural consequences are very likely to differ (see Nitsche & Paulus, 2000, for discussion on motor cortical function). For example, unlike TMS, tDCS does not "stimulate" neurons; rather the effects are due to modification of ongoing activity. While TMS pulses depolarise axons and generate action potentials, tDCS effects are sub-threshold and occur via polarisation of the resting membrane potential. Anodal tDCS typically has an excitatory neuronal effect due to a shift towards neuronal depolarisation, while cathodal stimulation elicits a hyperpolarisation (Bindman, Lippold, & Redfearn, 1962; Nitsche & Paulus, 2000; Purpura & McMurtry, 1965). Indeed, recent evidence suggests that tDCS polarises the resting membrane potential through the modulation of sodium and calcium dependent channels and NMDA-receptor activity (Nitsche et al., 2004; see Stagg & Nitsche, 2011, for a comprehensive review of pharmacological intervention to explore the mechanism of tDCS), thereby increasing or decreasing the mean firing rate of the neuron and promoting mechanisms of long-term potentiation and long-term depression (LTP/LTD) (Liebetanz, Nitsche, Tergau, & Paulus, 2002; Nitsche, Fricke, et al., 2003). Furthermore, an increased secretion of brain-derived neurotrophic factor (BDNF), a protein essential for new learning, has been associated with anodal stimulation (Fritsch et al., 2010). If we are to induce long-term consolidation, or the re-learning of information—a goal of aphasia therapy—a neuromodulatory method that has features of LTP-like processes is attractive.

Another attractive feature of tDCS is the apparent lack of any significant side effects. Large-scale cohort testing from different research centres has reported the most common adverse sensation is a slight itching sensation under the electrode and seldom-occurring headache, fatigue, and nausea (see Nitsche et al., 2008, Table 1; Poreisz, Boros, Antal, & Paulus, 2007). Although reports of skin burns associated with tDCS have been reported (Frank et al., 2011; Lagopoulos & Degabriele, 2008; Palm et al., 2008), these occurred in the context of extended stimulation periods (30 minutes), drying of electro-conductive gel, abraded skin surface, and the use of tap water to soak the sponge sheaths respectively. When conventional tDCS protocols were employed (i.e., 1–2 mA stimulation for up to 20 minutes), using optimised safety protocols, significant adverse effects, such as burning of the skin (Dundas, Thickbroom, & Mastaglia, 2007; Loo et al., 2011; Minhas et al., 2010) or heating of the electrodes and scalp surface (Datta, Elwassif, & Bikson, 2009; Nitsche & Paulus, 2000, 2001), were avoided. Under these protocol guidelines, tDCS may be considered safe (Nitsche, Schauenburg, et al., 2003). Furthermore, tDCS has not been reported to provoke seizures in non-acute neurological deficits, i.e., intervention protocols are well below the threshold of tissue damage (Liebetanz et al., 2009; Nitsche, Schauenburg, et al., 2003). Therefore, compared with TMS, tDCS may be a viable option for stimulation of perilesional cortex where the threshold to induce seizures is lower. In a clinical context this makes tDCS an appealing form of neurostimulation in chronic stroke populations (Priori, Hallett, & Rothwell, 2009). However, further investigation of tDCS hazards is certainly warranted in non-acute patients, both for existing protocols and those under development (Bikson, Datta, & Elwassif, 2009). In particular, the interaction of stimulation with different disease aetiologies and potential risk factors of seizure, such as lack of sleep (Nitsche et al., 2008)—as the propensity for seizure is much higher in acute and subacute patients. Therefore appropriate safety criteria are unknown, especially in the context of repeated protocols that may be required for rehabilitation.

Despite these caveats the technology is easy to use, relatively inexpensive, and portable, allowing treatment to be delivered not only in clinical settings but also in the patient's own home. tDCS is also well suited to online application; i.e., brain stimulation concurrent with behavioural intervention. For example, inferior frontal cortex (Broca's area) can be easily and comfortably targeted with tDCS. At the start of stimulation, most participants will perceive a slight itching sensation under the electrodes, which then quickly fades in most cases. In contrast, TMS and in particular rTMS, of the same region can inadvertently stimulate the trigeminal facial nerves causing facials twitches, or painful sensations making certain online tasks, such as spoken picture naming, very difficult. Therefore, for a treatment study that requires multiple sessions, TMS and repetitive TMS may be a less-suitable option. For research purposes it is also easier to conduct placebo (sham) stimulation-controlled studies with tDCS, because, with the exception of a slight itching sensation and mild sensory phenomena (including retinal phosphenes associated with current switching), participants rarely experience sensations related to the stimulation (Gandiga, Hummel, & Cohen, 2006). Therefore reliable effects of stimulation in the absence of any confounding "placebo effects" (i.e., the influence of participants' expectation of an effect on the observed results) may be achieved using tDCS.

Due to its appeal as a potential treatment tool, some manufacturers (NeuroConn, Germany, personal communication) are exploring mini-tDCS kits for patient's self-administration at home with stimulation dosages pre-programmed by their clinician. Some additional precautions should be considered for safe use of tDCS: (i) patients should have no metallic implants near the electrodes, and (ii) personnel conducting tDCS should be appropriately trained before applying the technique, as experience with the method is still limited and the risk profile of stimulation is not yet completely known. In the future, if successful, one could envisage a home treatment programme that the speech therapist would design involving concurrent tDCS with, e.g., a computer-delivered aphasia treatment programme.

tDCS AND REHABILITATION OF APHASIC STROKE PATIENTS

Two approaches have primarily been used in the application of cortical stimulation (tDCS and TMS) to rehabilitation of post-stroke aphasic patients. Both approaches to language recovery are based on a model of interhemispheric rivalry between the residual speech areas in the stroke-damaged left hemisphere and intact, non-stroke, right hemisphere (akin to models of motor recovery after stroke). In essence, the model proposes that speech deficits are due to (1) reduced output from the stroke-damaged left hemisphere and (2) excess inhibition of the left hemisphere from the intact, non-stroke, right hemisphere. Thus improvement may be possible either by increasing the output of the perilesional left hemisphere or decreasing the output from the intact, non-stroke, right hemisphere. In simple terms this could be achieved by using cortical stimulation to increase the excitability of the residual left hemisphere cortices or decrease the excitability of the intact right hemisphere (see Lindenberg, Renga, Zhu, Nair, & Schlaug, 2010; Vines, Cerruti, & Schlaug, 2008; both studies used bi-hemispheric stimulation to increase/decrease left and right cortical excitability). Despite the potential application of tDCS for language rehabilitation, to date just four studies in post-stroke aphasic patients have been reported (see Table 1). All of these studies aimed to improve speech production deficits by modulating the left hemisphere. The first study focused on the effects of a single session of stimulation applied to left frontal cortex (Monti et al., 2008). More recent work has emphasised the long-term effects on speech function that occur after repeated stimulation of left frontal or temporal cortices (Baker, Rorden, & Fridriksson, 2010; Fiori et al., 2010; Fridriksson, Richardson, Baker, & Rorden, 2011). We discuss each approach in turn below.

Single-session studies

The rationale behind these studies is to test if a single application of tDCS induces immediate gain in the selected outcome measures. At the same time these studies provide information about the safety and comfort of the intervention protocol. tDCS paradigms involving healthy speakers have typically used single-exposure approaches. That is, on a given session of tDCS a participant is exposed to anodal, cathodal, or sham stimulation for a relatively short period of time (e.g., 20 minutes) and their performance on language tasks is monitored. Tasks have included verbal fluency (Iyer et al., 2005), picture naming (Fertonani, Rosini, Cotelli, Rossini, & Miniussi, 2010; Sparing, Dafotakis, Hesse, & Fink, 2007), proper name retrieval (Ross, McCoy, Wolk, Coslett, & Olson, 2010), nonword–picture matching (Fiori et al., 2010; Liuzzi et al., 2010) and a wide range of designs, tDCS protocols and sites of stimulation were used. The evidence to date suggests that anodal relative to sham stimulation applied to the left hemisphere language cortices can significantly enhance normal language performance as measured by reaction time or accuracy.

Ideally, when applied to post-stroke aphasic patients, the gain should not just be greater than the effect of placebo (sham), or a traditional intervention, e.g., anomia treatment, but should also be of clinical significance. Although a satisfactory definition of clinical significance is difficult, most investigators would be content with an improvement of around 10% in standard aphasia measures, especially in the chronic stage post-stroke. Monti and colleagues (2008) used a single-session approach to assess change in post-stroke aphasic patients' picture-naming abilities. Eight chronic non-fluent aphasic patients took part in two sessions of tDCS separated by at least a week. In one session half of the patients received 2 mA anodal stimulation for 10 minutes applied to left fronto-temporal cortex immediately before a picture-naming task (i.e., offline). During the second session patients received sham stimulation applied to the same cortical region prior to picture naming. For the remaining patients, the intervention procedure was identical except that cathodal stimulation was delivered. The order of stimulation (anodal or cathodal) and sham was counterbalanced across sessions and patients. In contrast to the facilitatory results for anodal stimulation reported in the healthy participant literature, Monti and colleagues found an improvement in naming accuracy for cathodal stimulation in the order of 10.6%, with no significant effects after anodal and sham stimulation. This apparent paradoxical improvement in naming accuracy was argued to be due to a tDCS-induced depression of cortical inhibitory inter-neurons in the lesioned hemisphere, which led to a disinhibition of the cortex thereby improving the functioning of the damaged language cortices. Independent of the neural mechanisms, which remain elusive, this study indicated that it is possible to improve performance on a language task by means of a single dose of tDCS applied to the damaged left hemisphere. Subsequent tDCS and aphasia studies have aimed to investigate whether these intriguing naming improvements could be made to persist over an extended period of time.

Multiple-session studies

The hypothesis underlying multiple-session studies is that the short-lasting effects from a single session will accumulate with repeated sessions and eventually lead to a permanent improvement in function. Precisely how this approach might lead to a permanent improvement in language function in aphasic speakers after stroke is not clear. One possibility is that increasing the output from the stroke-damaged, left hemisphere will lead to more effective relearning of language. In other words, brain stimulation itself would not produce any lasting changes in language function; instead it would temporarily create a state that optimises relearning and rehabilitation. This natural process would lead to an improvement in language function and reduction in aphasic deficits. In healthy participants multiple sessions of left-sided anodal stimulation can improve overall performance when learning new information and associations relative to sham (e.g., de Vries et al., 2010; e.g., Fiori et al., 2010; Floël, Rosser, Miichka, Knecht, & Breitenstein, 2008). For language learning, a recent study applied anodal stimulation to left Broca's area online during the acquisition phase of an artificial grammar and demonstrated enhanced performance at detecting syntactic violations along with an increased use of rule-based decision making (de Vries et al., 2010). Similarly, anodal stimulation applied to left Wernicke's area during acquisition of an artificial lexicon increased the rate and overall success of language learning compared to sham stimulation after a single exposure to tDCS (Floël et al., 2008).

In relatively well-recovered aphasic patients, as in normal individuals, successful speech production has been correlated with brain activity in the stroke-damaged left hemisphere (Fridriksson, Bonilha, Baker, Moser, & Rorden, 2010). In this context, the interhemispheric model would predict that facilitating the remaining left perilesional cortex with excitatory stimulation could improve speech recovery (see Figure 2 later). Three tDCS studies (see Table 1) adopted this approach using a repeated intervention protocol that spanned several days with anodal tDCS delivered during a given task. This approach has been influenced, at least in part, by (i) the facilitatory effects observed in single-exposure studies of healthy participants and (ii) the idea that the favourable effects of mass-practice seen in behaviour-only anomia treatments may also be valid in combined tDCS and behavioural training approaches. Preliminary results suggest that anodal tDCS applied to the lesioned left hemisphere can facilitate naming performance post-treatment.

In the first treatment study 10 aphasic speakers were trained for five consecutive days using a spoken word-to-picture match task during which they received 20 minutes of anodal (1 mA) or sham stimulation of left frontal and precentral cortex

(Baker et al., 2010). The patients' naming accuracy improved on average by 8.4% after anodal stimulation compared to sham. Furthermore, improvements in naming were retained for at least 1 week for items that had been treated. Consistent with the behavioural rehabilitation literature, the observed facilitatory effects did not generalise to untreated items matched for psycholinguistic complexity. In a second study by this group the same treatment paradigm was used in eight mild fluent aphasic patients with lesions restricted to left posterior cortical and subcortical regions. Anodal stimulation was applied to left posterior perilesional cortex (Fridriksson et al., 2011) and as accuracy for naming was high at baseline in these patients, the outcome measure was reaction time. Anodal stimulation resulted in faster naming responses compared to sham stimulation. This naming improvement in the order of 38.2% faster persisted for at least three weeks. Again, the facilitatory effect of anodal stimulation was restricted to the treated items only. In the third study, Fiori and colleagues (2010) trained three non-fluent aphasic patients to name 80 pictures they could comprehend but not accurately produce. During naming practice 40 pictures were paired with 1 mA of anodal tDCS applied to left Wernicke's area and 40 pictures with sham stimulation of the same region. Anodal tDCS significantly improved naming accuracy by 20.5% on average compared to sham after 5 days of intervention.

DISCUSSION

Results from these first studies demonstrate, at the very least, that tDCS applied to the stroke-damaged left hemisphere in chronic aphasic patients is in principle (1) safe, there were no reported side effects reported in any of the studies, (2) well tolerated even when given over multiple sessions, and (3) can significantly modulate change in speech performance and relearning (see Figure 1 for schematic of mean percentage change

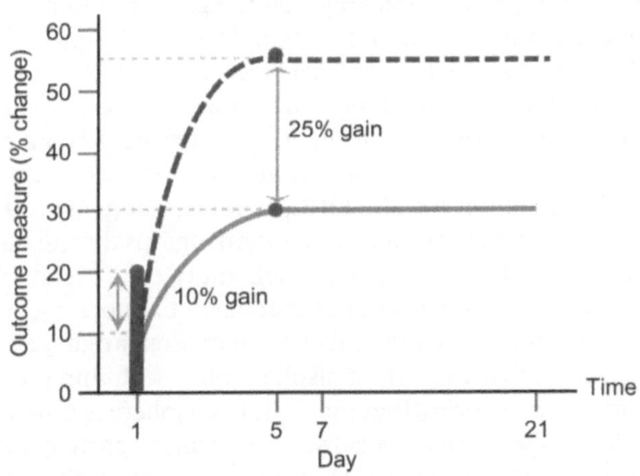

Figure 1. Summary schematic representation of potential tDCS effects in language performance in relation to normal re-learning after single and repeated interventions protocols (related to Table 1). Solid green line represents normal re-learning curve. Solid vertical red line indicates the potential percentage change in performance that may occur after a single intervention of tDCS. Dashed red line indicates potential performance change over 5 days from repeated tDCS delivered concurrently with treatment. Normal and tDCS-enhanced learning share an equivalent learning profile, however resulting gains post-tDCS may be modified by approximately 25%, with the effects of tDCS persisting for up to 3 weeks. To view this figure in colour, please see the online issue of the Journal.

in performance over time based on studies of language reviewed here). However, with such preliminary data a number of factors and questions emerge that may be key to understanding and developing tDCS as a truly adjuvant therapy tool in language recovery after aphasic stroke. The aim of this section is to discuss how to modify cortical excitability by tDCS with special emphasis on three methodological aspects. The first, *Where to stimulate*, considers the optimal site of stimulation in aphasic stroke patients and the role of the ipsilesional and contralesional hemispheres in supporting language rehabilitation. The second, *When to stimulate*, considers whether tDCS delivered before language rehabilitation (offline) or concurrently with the language task (online) may be most effective. The third, *How long to stimulate*, concerns the durations of tDCS intervention protocols. We discuss each in turn below. However, it is also important to emphasise that tDCS applied to aphasia research is in its early stages and therefore future studies might change some of the current concepts.

Where to stimulate

Identifying cortical regions to target with tDCS. The aim of current stimulation protocols is modulation of task-relevant regions of cortex. For tDCS to successfully modulate a component of an intact or impaired language system, the brain regions that support a given task must first be identified. Functional magnetic resonance imaging (fMRI) has been extensively used to explore which regions of the brain are associated with a variety of different language tasks. In the case of speech production meta-analyses revealed that a large, predominantly left-lateralised perisylvian network is involved. Depending on the task delivered during scanning, the extended speech production network is differentially engaged (for review see Price, 2010; Vigneau et al., 2006) with frontal (de Zubicaray & McMahon, 2009; Fridriksson et al., 2009; Papoutsi et al., 2009), premotor, motor (Brown et al., 2009), or posterior temporal (Abel et al., 2009; Hocking, McMahon, & de Zubicaray, 2009) regions predominantly activated.

In an attempt to determine the key, or functionally critical, regions within these language networks identified by fMRI, researchers have used TMS and rTMS. For example, in healthy speakers TMS "virtual lesion" methods have been applied to determine the involvement of (i) frontal regions during action naming (Cappa et al., 2002) and repetition priming (Thiel et al., 2005); (ii) left anterior temporal regions during verb generation (Holland & Lambon Ralph, 2010), synonym judgement (Pobric, Jefferies, & Lambon Ralph, 2007); and left posterior temporal regions during object recognition (Stewart, Meyer, Frith, & Rothwell, 2001). Each study used results from functional neuroimaging to inform the stimulation site that when temporarily "lesioned" by the TMS protocols would determine its relevance for a chosen language task.

While the consensus is that the left hemisphere plays a dominant role in language processing, it is worth remembering that the right hemisphere is also significantly activated in a range of language tasks. A recent study of healthy participants used fMRI to guide rTMS to target the right posterior inferior frontal gyrus (IFG) during phonological decisions on words (Hartwigsen et al., 2010). They found that TMS applied over the left, right, or bilateral IFG disrupted phonological processing to an equivalent degree. This suggests that the left and right IFG do not have the capacity to rapidly compensate for disruption to the other during rTMS in healthy participants. However, in chronic post-stroke aphasia the interhemispheric relationship may be altered as a consequence of time and brain–language recovery after stroke. Understanding these patterns of variation may be key factors in developing more sophisticated models of language processing and recovery that will, in turn, inform suitable target sites for stimulation in aphasic patients.

Identifying viable cortex to stimulate in damaged brains. When translating stimulation protocols from healthy participants to post-stroke aphasic patients, the consideration is not only in terms of how the stimulation target site may be engaged by the language task, but also how the stroke damage impacts on the targeted cortical region's structure and function. In the four studies reviewed here, two used each patient's own fMRI brain activation patterns collected during overt picture naming to subsequently guide the placement of tDCS electrodes (Baker et al., 2010; Fridriksson et al., 2011) while the remaining two studies were guided by data from previous neuroimaging studies.

In each study the active electrode was placed directly over the cortex to be modulated, as the electrical field strength induced by tDCS decreases rapidly with distance from the electrode (Miranda, Lomarev, & Hallett, 2006). However, the placement of the active electrode on the scalp varied across the four studies reviewed here. They included primarily left frontal (Baker et al., 2010) and left temporal regions (Fiori et al., 2010; Fridriksson et al., 2011; Monti et al., 2008). Baker et al. (2010) found that, across their group of patients with frontal or posterior lesions, those who showed the greatest improvement in naming accuracy after frontal anodal tDCS were those with perilesional areas closest to the electrode site. Indeed, in a more homogeneous group of patients, seven out of eight patients with posterior cortical or subcortical lesions showed faster naming responses after posterior anodal tDCS (Fridriksson et al., 2011), again highlighting the role of perilesional regions in supporting language processes. In the study by Fiori and colleagues (2010) they noted that the lesion of one of their patients, M.T., completely overlapped with the electrode location, yet surprisingly this patient also showed an improvement in naming accuracy by the fifth day of treatment in the order of ~7% relative to sham. These results suggest that the cortical effect of tDCS in this patient must be remote from the electrode site, but how this is mediated is unclear.

Using the model of interhemispheric rivalry, if speech production performance is to be successfully improved after partial left hemisphere stroke damage then anodal tDCS applied to structurally and/or functionally intact perilesional cortex should increase the residual left hemisphere's output and improve language function. Indeed, both Baker et al., (2010) and Fridriksson et al., (2011) have used this approach. Here functioning perilesional left hemisphere cortex was identified using fMRI pre-treatment to ensure that tDCS was delivered to both functionally and structurally viable cortical tissue. However, if suitable cortex in the stroke-damaged left hemisphere were not available due to an extensive lesion for example, an alternative approach to treatment would be necessary. Again, based on the model of interhemispheric rivalry, in such cases tDCS could be applied to the right hemisphere to enhance residual output from the stroke-damaged hemisphere by removing any potential interference, or reducing the excitability of the right hemisphere i.e., inhibitory stimulation of the contralesional, right hemisphere (see Figure 2).

Stimulation of the contralesional hemisphere as a method of suppressing the maladaptive strategies of the unaffected hemisphere and promoting activity of the damaged hemisphere has been explored in the context of motor recovery post-stroke. Results indicate that, like positive effects observed for anodal stimulation of the ipsilesional hemisphere, cathodal stimulation of the contralesional hemisphere also

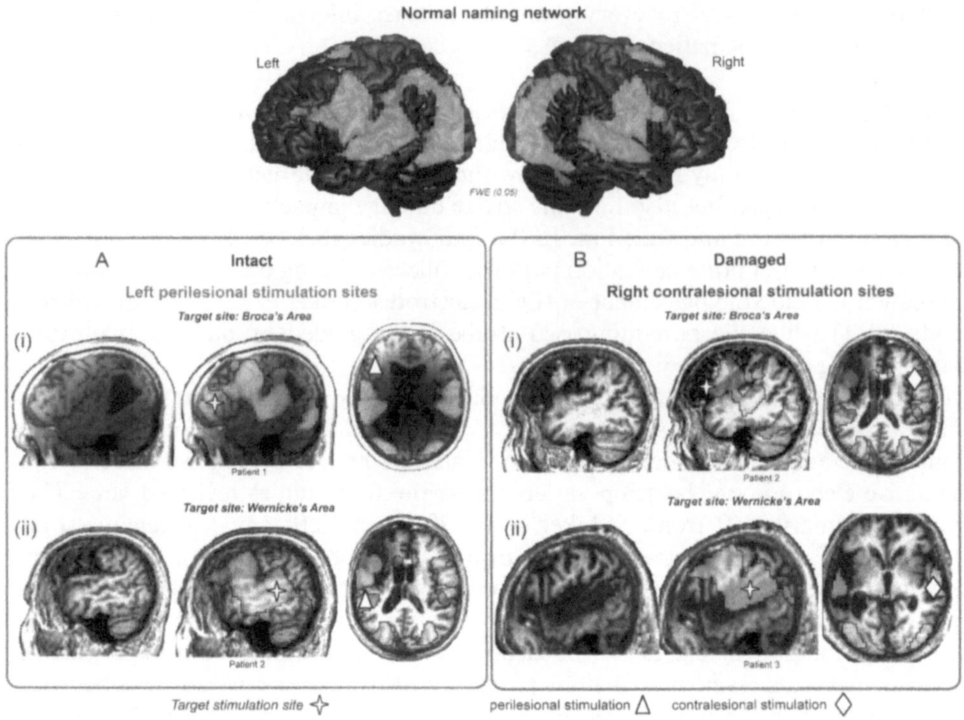

Figure 2. Illustration of potential target sites of stimulation to facilitate naming performance in relation to structural brain damage and the normal naming network in three different patients. The top panel illustrates the extensive bilateral fronto-temporal naming network found in an fMRI study of healthy older particpants (cf. Holland et al., 2011). Activation is overlaid onto a rendered cortical surface from SPM8. In the lower panels of the figure we overlay the normal pattern of brain activation onto three chronic aphasic stroke patients' individual structural MRI scans. The aim here is to illustrate from left to right for each patient: (1) their structural brain damage within the left hemisphere, (2) the normal naming network overlaid onto their individual brain scan to show the relationship between the lesion damage to the naming network and the target stimulation site (red cross), and (3) the stimulation sites feasible for each patient depending on the proposed target site. Panel A highlights, in two chronic aphasic stroke patients, that structurally intact regions of cortex within the lesioned left hemisphere may serve as potential candidate sites for anodal stimulation to facilitate treatment of anomia in (Ai) Broca's area and (Aii) Wernicke's area. Panel B highlights that when the lesion is has damaged relevant cortices in the left hemisphere perilesional stimulation may not be possible. Therefore, for the two patients illustrated, facilitation of the contralesional hemisphere may be the optimal approach to aid recovery: (Bi) right homologue to Broca's area and (Bii) Wernicke's area. Although not illustrated here, in cases where patients have suffered a large MCA infarct affecting the whole of the left hemisphere and resulted in extremely limited perilesional tissue, stimulation of the contralesional hemisphere would be the sole option. Furthermore, studies of aphasia recovery have successfully used anodal stimulation of the left perilesional hemisphere to elicit positive behavioural outcomes, however the effects of anodal or cathodal stimulation of the right contralesional hemisphere are, as yet unknown, and will be dependent on the theoretical hypotheses of the research. To view this figure in colour, please see the online issue of the Journal.

enhanced motor performance (Boggio et al., 2007; Fregni et al., 2005). Furthermore, bi-hemispheric stimulation of the left and right hemisphere with anodal and cathodal in healthy participants enhanced motor performance to a greater degree than unilateral or sham stimulation (Vines et al., 2008). This pattern of improved performance following "dual" stimulation was replicated in a group of 10 chronic stoke patients compared to a group of 10 patients who received sham stimulation (Lindenberg et al., 2010), suggesting preliminary support for this approach.

Surprisingly, such an electrode arrangement has not yet been used in tDCS studies of language recovery in post-stroke aphasic patients. While in the TMS literature stimulation of the contralesional hemisphere as a method of suppressing the maladaptive strategies of the right, non-lesioned hemisphere during language tasks and thereby promoting activity of the lesioned hemisphere has been the main approach to date (Hamilton, Chrysikou, & Coslett, 2011). Functional neuroimaging studies have shown chronic over-activation of the non-dominant language homologues (Blank, Bird, Turkheimer, & Wise, 2003; Leff et al., 2002; Naeser et al., 2004; Rosen et al., 2000), especially in severely aphasic patients (Crinion & Price, 2005). In the case of speech production it is hypothesised that suppressive stimulation over the right frontal cortices (homologue to Broca's area) would promote the recovery of speech function. Naeser et al., (2005) found such an effect in four chronic patients of variable severity when given 10 daily sessions of 1 Hz rTMS over the right hemisphere homologue of Broca's area. The patients had an immediate improvement in picture naming output that, for three patients, persisted for up to 8 months.

In contrast, a later study by Winhuisen and colleagues (2005) showed that verbal fluency could be significantly reduced after stimulation of the right inferior frontal gyrus (IFG). They studied 11 patients within 2 weeks of their stroke and applied 4 Hz rTMS over the right IFG for 10 seconds during a verbal fluency task. Pre-treatment positron emission tomography (PET) showed that eight patients showed activation of the right IFG during this task and, in five of these patients, fluency was reduced by stimulation of the right IFG. The conclusion from this study was that in some patients activity in the right IFG at least in this early time post stroke was contributing to speech rather than interfering with function of Broca's area on the left. These data highlight the issue of general applicability of a treatment approach using suppression of the non-stroke hemisphere; for a subset of these patients the right IFG was also essential for residual language function. Therefore the preliminary results from tDCS of the right hemisphere to promote motor recovery are encouraging (e.g., Lindenberg et al., 2010; Vines et al., 2008), but more research is needed to explore whether these issues of individual differences that apply to TMS effects of the motor cortex may also apply for tDCS of the language cortices.

Furthermore, Martin and colleagues (2004), using a single session of 1 Hz rTMS under magnetic resonance imaging navigation, showed that the nature of the stimulation effect may depend on the exact site of stimulation: picture naming was transiently improved by rTMS only after suppression of the anterior portion of the IFG (Broca's area), whereas stimulation of the posterior parts of Broca's area had the opposite effect. If cognitive models predict subtle gradations within proximal cortical regions, an issue that is particularly problematic for tDCS is spatial specificity within a target stimulation site, which may preclude its use to explore such empirical questions. We discuss this issue in the following section.

tDCS focality. While TMS has been successfully used in exploring subtle spatial variation across different cortical regions (Devlin, Matthews, & Rushworth, 2003; Gough, Nobre, & Devlin, 2005; Nixon, Lazarova, Hodinott-Hill, Gough, & Passingham, 2004) tDCS is argued to lack such spatial specificity due to (a) using large electrodes and (b) the bipolar scalp electrode arrangement used in many studies. Electrodes are typically quite large, ranging from 25–35cm^2, therefore tDCS may stimulate not only the intended cortex, but also adjacent cortices. This limits the use of tDCS for detailed anatomical mapping and differential stimulation of cortical regions in close proximity to one another. As such, the issue of focality remains an important consideration in brain stimulation studies and may preclude the use of tDCS in favour of (r)TMS to explore certain research questions. However, to increase the focality of tDCS, researchers are investigating different electrode geometries (Datta, Bansal, et al., 2009) and reducing the size of the electrodes, while maintaining the level of direct current delivered. For example, it has been shown that a smaller ($3.5cm^2$) electrode and reduced current 0.1 mA induced equivalent effects on cortico-spinal activity (Nitsche, Doemkes, et al., 2007). However, the effects of smaller electrodes on tissue excitability due to changes in current orientation and edge effects, for example, are unclear and require further development and investigation highlighting that the solution is not a simple one (Nitsche et al., 2008).

Another consideration of tDCS is that, by definition, it relies on delivering current via electrodes placed on the scalp surface (transcranially). It has been suggested that much of the current delivered is shunted through the scalp, with only half of an injected current entering the cortex (Miranda et al., 2006). The electrical field strength induced by tDCS also decreases rapidly with distance from the electrode, which may preclude the use of tDCS to target deep cortical structures, such as the insula, in speech production tasks in healthy and impaired speakers.

When deciding where to stimulate with tDCS, there is also the question of where to place the reference electrode. All tDCS protocols require that there are two electrodes between which a direct, constant current must flow from the anode (positively charged) to the cathode (negatively charged). In paradigms that refer to anodal or cathodal stimulation effects the second "reference" electrode is located over an area deemed to be remote from cortical regions involved in the task. In tDCS studies of language processing to date, the location of the reference electrode has varied from contralateral supraorbital ridge (Fiori et al., 2010; Liuzzi et al., 2010), vertex (Sparing et al., 2007), the cheekbone (Ross et al., 2010), to an extracephalic site (Baker et al., 2010; Fertonani et al., 2010; Fridriksson et al., 2011; Monti et al., 2008). Issues arise concerning each montage of electrodes. If both electrodes are placed on the scalp (bi-cephalic montage), it has been argued that observed tDCS effects may be due to a combination of facilitation and/or inhibition across the brain, giving rise to a widespread change of cortical excitability (Lang et al., 2005). However, making inferences about the source of tDCS effects is difficult. Although this is an important consideration, evidence from the motor-tDCS literature suggests that neurobehavioural measures of excitability of the motor cortex (e.g., motor evoked potentials) are unaffected by a supraorbital reference electrode (Nitsche & Paulus, 2000). To further address such concerns, another approach has been to use an enlarged reference electrode relative to the active electrode. A large reference electrode renders the current too dispersed to be effective (current density = current strength divided by the electrode size)—therefore making the reference electrode stimulation theoretically neutral—allowing for the inference that the observed effects on brain and behaviour are solely due to modulation of the target cortex by the active electrode. Research in the motor literature indicates that tDCS effects were equivalent across the standard and enlarged electrode geometries (Nitsche, Doemkes, et al., 2007).

Avoiding any potential confounding effects of two electrodes with opposite polarities over the brain, an extracephalic reference was used in two of the tDCS studies in this review (e.g., Baker et al., 2010; Fridriksson et al., 2011). In motor studies this electrode arrangement has been suggested to allow for potential spinal influence on observed effects via cortico-spinal connections (e.g., Nitsche, Doemkes, et al., 2007). However, a recent study exploring autonomic responses to anodal, cathodal, and sham stimulation of the frontal midline with an extracephalic reference found no significant effects of stimulation with an extra-cephalic reference (Vandermeeren, Jamart, & Ossemann, 2010). It is important to note that at this stage it is not clear which is the "best" approach to use, but any differences in the arrangement of electrode may influence effects of stimulation (Miranda et al., 2006) and should therefore be clearly reported to allow for comparison across studies (cf. Nitsche et al., 2008).

When to stimulate. As with TMS, an important empirical question is when to deliver tDCS in relation to a task of interest, i.e., online: concurrently with the task or offline: pre-task (at rest). The choice depends on the hypotheses about the neural mechanisms supporting the behavioural effects. To date, the neural mechanisms that support tDCS remain unclear (Nitsche, Fricke, et al., 2003; Nitsche, Liebetanz, et al., 2003; Nitsche & Paulus, 2000).

The offline approach uses tDCS to prime the system at rest in preparation for a task to be performed after stimulation. It has been successfully used in language studies of both healthy (Fertonani et al., 2010) and impaired speakers (Monti et al., 2008). In contrast to Fertonani and colleagues, who report an improvement in performance after offline anodal tDCS, Monti et al. found an improvement in patients' naming accuracy after offline cathodal stimulation of left fronto-temporal cortex. This apparent contradictory effect observed for cathodal rather than anodal stimulation was argued to be due to tDCS-induced depression of cortical inhibitory inter-neurons in the lesioned hemisphere. This in turn led to a disinhibition of the cortex, thereby improving the function of the damaged left hemisphere language areas. This paradoxical improvement has also been reported in a motion detection study (Antal, Nitsche, Kruse, et al., 2004). Further research using offline stimulation to precondition the cortex prior to delivery of a task is certainly needed in order to better understand these contrasting effects.

In contrast, several studies have used online tDCS delivered during a language task (Iyer et al., 2005; Ross et al., 2010; Sparing et al., 2007), and during language learning in healthy participants (de Vries et al., 2010; Fiori et al., 2010; Floël et al., 2008). Consistent with the approach of these latter studies the facilitatory effects of anodal stimulation on motor learning was found to be maximal when delivered during motor skill training. In contrast, tDCS applied at rest, i.e., not paired with training, had no beneficial effect on motor performance (Nitsche, Roth, et al., 2007; Nitsche, Schauenburg, et al., 2003).

At a cellular and molecular level, studies in basic science suggest that one possible neurobiological account of the mechanism underlying the facilitatory effects of online anodal stimulation is that during anodal tDCS the intracellular calcium concentrations, which are important for processes of LTP, are increased via improved transmembrane calcium conduction (Canepari, Djurisic, & Zecevic, 2007). Furthermore, there is an increased secretion of brain-derived neurotrophic factor (BDNF), a protein crucial for new learning that occurs during anodal stimulation (Fritsch et al., 2010). Conversely, anodal modulation of synaptic strength prior to motor learning has been shown to compromise performance (Kuo et al., 2008), an effect that was further modulated by the presence of a partial NMDA-receptor agonist (d-cycloserine). Similarly, the enhancement of motor cortex excitability by preconditioning with anodal tDCS elicited decreased excitation in rTMS protocols that had previously had no effect (Siebner et al., 2004). The excitability status, or homeostatic plasticity, of the underlying cortex is important as it modulates the ease with which synaptic connections can be facilitated or suppressed (e.g., Antal, Terney, Poreisz, & Paulus, 2007).

Increased excitability within a language-engaged network (during practice or therapy) and the associated neurobiological facilitation of cellular and molecular mechanisms of anodal tDCS may together have the capacity for increased neuroplasticity within the damaged language system, which may increase the potential for better learning or language recovery. Specifically, within a task-engaged network the synchronous firing of post-synaptic targets will encourage synaptic strengthening (Kuo et al., 2008; Nitsche, Roth, et al., 2007). Therefore, it could be argued that in the context of re-learning language and aphasia therapy tDCS delivered during, and not before, a task or learning paradigm could optimise outcome and long-term language performance. Although preconditioning—or offline stimulation—of the cortex with tDCS has been shown to enhance subsequent neural effects of TMS (e.g., Lang et al., 2004; Siebner et al., 2004), the comparison of offline and online tDCS stimulation protocols, their effect on behavioural performance and relationship to the underlying neural mechanism of tDCS requires further systematic research.

How long to stimulate. The efficacy of tDCS from current density and stimulation duration has been systematically explored in the primary motor cortex. Increasing current density or stimulation duration, holding the other parameter constant, results in longer-lasting and stronger effects (Nitsche, Nitsche, et al., 2003; Nitsche & Paulus, 2000, 2001). However, this might not be a linear relationship in each case. Larger current densities also increase the depth of the electrical field modulating deeper cortical regions not affected by lower intensity protocols and where the effects of tDCS might be different compared with more superficial cortical structures (Creutzfeldt, Fromm, & Kapp, 1962). Moreover, large current densities might be painful. Current densities delivered during language studies have varied between 0.029 and 0.08 mA/cm^2 in most published studies (see Floël, 2012, and Table 1). These limits will probably continue to expand with experience (Nitsche et al., 2008).

Similarly, one might consider that repeated delivery of tDCS paired with repeated activation of a task-engaged network should be incrementally beneficial. However, stimulation durations, which are likely to result in excitability changes lasting more than 1 hour, should be applied with caution, because changes lasting that long could be consolidated and stabilised leading to unintended or adverse effects: i.e., beyond a certain period of time, the enhancing effects of anodal tDCS may switch and become inhibitory (Fricke et al., 2010). The same concerns apply for repeated application of tDCS to the same brain region without an appropriate interval between sessions (Monte-Silva et al., 2010). When repetitive tDCS is performed to prolong and stabilise long-lasting after-effects, participants are generally stimulated once a day (Boggio et al., 2007; Fregni et al., 2006). Although repeated interventions in the order of days appeared to give facilitatory effects on language performance in aphasic speakers (see Table 1), and language learning in healthy speakers (de Vries et al., 2010; Floël et al., 2008), it remains unclear whether this protocol is optimally suited to maximise the electrophysiological effects of tDCS.

At present, 20 minutes of anodal tDCS given within a session appears to be facilitatory, with the effects lasting at least as long as the duration of stimulation. However, beyond 20 minutes of stimulation the effects may not be as expected. For repeated application of tDCS, we suggest a sufficiently long intersession interval between tDCS interventions to avoid unintended carry-over effects. The duration of this interval depends on the stimulation procedure. If the aim is to induce more long-term and stable changes in cortical function, repeated daily tDCS sessions may be adequate. However, further studies are certainly needed to explore the optimal intersession interval for stabilising effects. So contrary to the general "more is better" approach for aphasia behavioural therapeutic interventions, this adage may not be the case with tDCS.

CAVEATS

Despite significant limitations to our understanding of the mechanism of tDCS, the preliminary work with chronic aphasic stroke patients reviewed here indicate that it is possible to improve language task performance by means of noninvasive electrical stimulation applied to the damaged brain. This raises the exciting hypothesis that currently available tDCS has the potential to modulate language rehabilitation. Several caveats should be kept in mind.

First, studies implemented so far have mostly focused on the ability of tDCS to elicit improvements in speech production by stimulation of left-hemisphere perilesional regions. Yet the accompanying neural mechanisms underlying these changes have not been investigated. The paths of tDCS-induced effects remain unclear and behavioural changes may result through specific enhancement of activity in the targeted cortical area or via distant effects on other interconnected cortical areas. Therefore more sophisticated head models incorporating detailed anatomical information from structural MRI or DTI may be necessary to constrain tDCS effects. At the very least in aphasic stroke patients a detailed anatomical MRI scan is necessary to be confident that the active electrode is placed over structurally intact cortex.

Second, detailed theoretical and anatomical models of language processing that guide the application of tDCS to particular regions of cortex are also necessary. fMRI and TMS studies of language processing have highlighted that the right hemisphere may well have a contributing role to play in aphasia recovery emphasising that therapeutic interventions, such as tDCS, that stress targeting the left or right-hemisphere currently should be based on supporting functional neuroimaging of patients and language tasks. Studies combining tDCS with other brain imaging and neurophysiologic mapping methods, e.g., fMRI or electroencephalography (EEG), promise to provide invaluable insights on the correlation between modification of language and its underlying neurophysiological mechanisms.

Third, most basic neuroscience research in the field has focused on studying the effects of stimulation over the motor cortex, where anodal stimulation has a facilitatory effect and cathodal an inhibitory effect. However, some studies have reported that anodal stimulation of the frontal cortex failed to induce significant improvements in behaviour (Antal, Nitsche, Kincses, et al., 2004; Nitsche, Schauenburg, et al., 2003). Similarly, cathodal tDCS does not always inhibit language performance in healthy participants (e.g., Fertonani et al., 2010; Iyer et al., 2005; Sparing et al., 2007). However, studies indicating a lack of effect of stimulation in a particular cortical region are not proof that that area is not involved. The most parsimonious interpretation of these findings is that more elaborate, hypothesis-driven behavioural paradigms or stimulation parameters may be necessary to study the functional role of the cortical regions involved in language processing. Alternatively, it is possible that the "threshold" for facilitating motor learning by stimulation of motor cortex is lower than by stimulation of other cortical areas for language processing, an issue that needs to be investigated in future experiments.

Finally, studies to date have focused on relatively short-term improvements in language performance (longest follow-up data available in aphasic patients was 3 weeks post training; Fridriksson et al., 2010). It is not known whether these intriguing task-specific improvements may be persistent or have any impact on real-life functional communication abilities. More experiments are required to assess the effects of repeated applications of tDCS in association with multiple training sessions, their interaction with specific language tasks and different intensive training regimes, such as constraint-induced aphasia treatment (CIAT) and the extent to which these performance improvements are retained in the long term. Therefore these factors should be considered when designing a study.

CONCLUSIONS AND FUTURE DIRECTIONS

In summary, despite the infancy of the field and the very few studies to date, it does seem possible to improve aphasic stroke patients' performance on speech production tasks by means of tDCS. The lack of any reported adverse effects suggests that the procedure is safe, even in chronic stroke patients who have a higher reported incidence of seizures than healthy participants. Future work will have to address many so-far unanswered questions including:

(1) *What are the optimal combinations of stimulation parameters to get maximal behavioural effects?* For tDCS these parameters involve the size of electrodes, amplitude, duration of current, online versus offline, and the time-interval between stimulation periods. A systematic exploration of how these parameters interact and influence tDCS-induced effects in normal language function is certainly important. How these effects then translate to damaged brains is an additional level of complexity that may also vary with time post-stroke. Furthermore, whether established tDCS protocols may be usefully combined with other forms of therapeutic intervention: for example pharmacological interventions also needs investigation. Pharmacotherapy for recovery from aphasia when delivered in combination with behavioural training (Berthier et al., 2009) may have maximal potential when also combined with tDCS. While drugs may have a more global effect on brain function, tDCS can have a more regionally specific effect (Holland et al., 2011). Therefore, when administered in combination with language rehabilitation, these approaches may have a synergistic effect. For example, tDCS of frontal cortex during speech production in combination with pharmacological modification of the dopaminergic system may enhance, or prolong, therapeutic outcome compared to each intervention alone (e.g., Antal & Paulus, 2011).

(2) *When applying tDCS to facilitate aphasia recovery is it more effective to stimulate the stroke-damaged or the non-stroke hemisphere?* Although the model of interhemispheric rivalry has been used to support the idea that excitatory tDCS should be applied to the stroke hemisphere to optimise recovery, the corollary argument that inhibition of the right hemisphere with tDCS is beneficial requires further research. As suggested by some TMS studies of interference with language function, it may well be that in some aphasic patients the right hemisphere is contributing significantly to their language recovery, rather than suppressing remaining function of the stroke hemisphere. In this instance these patients may benefit from anodal tDCS to

the right hemisphere: one approach may not be suitable for all. Further work is certainly needed to understand the mechanism of tDCS. Nevertheless, at this stage there is an encouraging possibility that tDCS of perilesional cortices when combined with behavioural rehabilitation may contribute to improved speech outcome in post-stroke aphasic patients. These preliminary foundations suggest that tDCS as a complementary tool for rehabilitation of language function in chronic stroke aphasic patients is an exciting opportunity and an important new avenue of research.

REFERENCES

Abel, S., Dressel, K., Bitzer, R., Kummerer, D., Mader, I., Weiller, C., et al. (2009). The separation of processing stages in a lexical interference fMRI-paradigm. *NeuroImage, 44*(3), 1113–1124.

Antal, A., Nitsche, M. A., Kincses, T. Z., Kruse, W., Hoffmann, K. P., & Paulus, W. (2004). Facilitation of visuo-motor learning by transcranial direct current stimulation of the motor and extrastriate visual areas in humans. *European Journal of Neuroscience, 19*(10), 2888–2892.

Antal, A., Nitsche, M. A., Kruse, W., Kincses, T. Z., Hoffmann, K. P., & Paulus, W. (2004). Direct current stimulation over V5 enhances visuomotor coordination by improving motion perception in humans. *Journal of Cognitive Neuroscience, 16*(4), 521–527.

Antal, A., & Paulus, W. (2011). A case of refractory orofacial pain treated by transcranial direct current stimulation applied over hand motor area in combination with NMDA agonist drug intake. *Brain Stimulation, 4*(2), 117–121.

Antal, A., Terney, D., Poreisz, C., & Paulus, W. (2007). Towards unravelling task-related modulations of neuroplastic changes induced in the human motor cortex. *European Journal of Neuroscience, 26*(9), 2687–2691.

Baker, J. M., Rorden, C., & Fridriksson, J. (2010). Using transcranial direct-current stimulation to treat stroke patients with aphasia. *Stroke, 41*(6), 1229–1236.

Barthel, G., Meinzer, M., Djundja, D., & Rockstroh, B. (2008). Intensive language therapy in chronic aphasia: Which aspects contribute most? *Aphasiology, 22*(4), 408–421.

Berthier, M. L., Green, C., Lara, J. P., Higueras, C., Barbancho, M. A., Davila, G., et al. (2009). Memantine and constraint-induced aphasia therapy in chronic poststroke aphasia. *Annals of Neurology, 65*(5), 577–585.

Bhogal, S. K., Teasell, R. W., Foley, N. C., & Speechley, M. R. (2003). Rehabilitation of aphasia: More is better. *Topics in Stroke Rehabilitation, 10*(2), 66–76.

Bikson, M., Datta, A., & Elwassif, M. (2009). Establishing safety limits for transcranial direct current stimulation. *Clinical Neurophysiology, 120*(6), 1033–1034.

Bindman, L. J., Lippold, O. C., & Redfearn, J. W. (1962). Long-lasting changes in the level of the electrical activity of the cerebral cortex produced bypolarizing currents. *Nature, 196*, 584–585.

Blank, S. C., Bird, H., Turkheimer, F., & Wise, R. J. (2003). Speech production after stroke: The role of the right pars opercularis. *Annals of Neurology, 54*(3), 310–320.

Boggio, P. S., Nunes, A., Rigonatti, S. P., Nitsche, M. A., Pascual-Leone, A., & Fregni, F. (2007). Repeated sessions of noninvasive brain DC stimulation is associated with motor function improvement in stroke patients. *Restorative Neurology and Neuroscience, 25*(2), 123–129.

Breitenstein, C., Kramer, K., Meinzer, M., Baumgartner, A., Floël, A., & Knecht, S. (2009). Intense language training for aphasia. Contribution of cognitive factors. *Nervenarzt, 80*(2), 149–150.

Brindley, P., Copeland, M., Demain, C., & Martyn, P. (1989). Comparison of the speech of ten chronic Broca's aphasics following intensive and nonintensive periods of therapy. *Aphasiology, 3*, 695–707.

Brown, S., Laird, A. R., Pfordresher, P. Q., Thelen, S. M., Turkeltaub, P., & Liotti, M. (2009). The somatotopy of speech: Phonation and articulation in the human motor cortex. *Brain and Cognition, 70*(1), 31–41.

Canepari, M., Djurisic, M., & Zecevic, D. (2007). Dendritic signals from rat hippocampal CA1 pyramidal neurons during coincident pre- and post-synaptic activity: A combined voltage- and calcium-imaging study. *Journal of Physiology, 580*, 463–484.

Cappa, S. F., Sandrini, M., Rossini, P. M., Sosta, K., & Miniussi, C. (2002). The role of the left frontal lobe in action naming – rTMS evidence. *Neurology, 59*(5), 720–723.

Cherney, L. R., Patterson, J. P., Raymer, A., Frymark, T., & Schooling, T. (2008). Evidence-based systematic review: Effects of intensity of treatment and constraint-induced language therapy for individuals with stroke-induced aphasia. *Journal of Speech, Language and Hearing Research, 51*(5), 1282–1299.

Cohen Kadosh, R., Soskic, S., Iuculano, T., Kanai, R., & Walsh, V. (2010). Modulating neuronal activity produces specific and long-lasting changes in numerical competence. *Current Biology, 20*, 1–5.

Creutzfeldt, O. D., Fromm, G. H., & Kapp, H. (1962). Influence of transcortical d-c currents on cortical neuronal activity. *Experimental Neurology, 5*, 436–452.

Crinion, J., & Price, C. J. (2005). Right anterior superior temporal activation predicts auditory sentence comprehension following aphasic stroke. *Brain, 128*(Pt 12), 2858–2871.

Datta, A., Bansal, V., Diaz, J., Patel, J., Reato, D., & Bikson, M. (2009). Gyri -precise head model of transcranial DC stimulation: Improved spatial focality using a ring electrode versus conventional rectangular pad. *Brain Stimulation, 2*(4), 201–207.

Datta, A., Elwassif, M., & Bikson, M. (2009). Bio-heat transfer model of transcranial DC stimulation: comparison of conventional pad versus ring electrode. *Conference proceedings: Annual International Conference of the IEEE Engineering in Medicine and Biology Society, 2009*, 670–673.

de Vries, M. H., Barth, A. C. R., Maiworm, S., Knecht, S., Zwitserlood, P., & Floël, A. (2010). Electrical stimulation of Broca's area enhances implicit learning of an artificial grammar. *Journal of Cognitive Neuroscience, 22*(11), 2427–2436.

de Zubicaray, G. I., & McMahon, K. L. (2009). Auditory context effects in picture naming investigated with event-related fMRI. *Cognitive Affective and Behavioral Neuroscience, 9*(3), 260–269.

Devlin, J. T., Matthews, P. M., & Rushworth, M. F. (2003). Semantic processing in the left inferior prefrontal cortex: A combined functional magnetic resonance imaging and transcranial magnetic stimulation study. *Journal of Neuroscience, 15*(1), 71–84.

Dockery, C. A., Hueckel-Weng, R., Birbaumer, N., & Plewnia, C. (2009). Enhancement of planning ability by transcranial direct current stimulation. *Journal of Neuroscience, 29*(22), 7271–7277.

Dundas, J. E., Thickbroom, G. W., & Mastaglia, F. L. (2007). Perception of comfort during transcranial DC stimulation: Effect of NaCl solution concentration applied to sponge electrodes. *Clinical Neurophysiology, 118*(5), 1166–1170.

Fertonani, A., Rosini, S., Cotelli, M., Rossini, P. M., & Miniussi, C. (2010). Naming facilitation induced by transcranial direct current stimulation. *Behavioral Brain Research, 208*(2), 311–318.

Fiori, V., Coccia, M., Marinelli, C. V., Vecchi, V., Bonifazi, S., Ceravolo, M. G., et al. (2010). Transcranial direct current stimulation improves word retrieval in healthy and nonfluent aphasic subjects. *Journal of Cognitive Neuroscience, 23*(9), 2309–2323.

Floël, A., Rosser, N., Miichka, O., Knecht, S., & Breitenstein, C. (2008). Noninvasive brain stimulation improves language learning. *Journal of Cognitive Neuroscience, 20*(8), 1415–1422.

Frank, E., Eichhammer, P., Burger, J., Zowe, M., Landgrebe, M., Hajak, G., et al. (2011). Transcranial magnetic stimulation for the treatment of depression: Feasibility and results under naturalistic conditions: A retrospective analysis. *European Archives of Psychiatry and Clinical Neuroscience, 261*(4), 261–266.

Fregni, F., Boggio, P. S., Lima, M. C., Ferreira, M. J., Wagner, T., Rigonatti, S. P., et al. (2006). A sham-controlled, phase II trial of transcranial direct current stimulation for the treatment of central pain in traumatic spinal cord injury. *Pain, 122*(1–2), 197–209.

Fregni, F., Boggio, P. S., Mansur, C. G., Wagner, T., Ferreira, M. J. L., Lima, M. C., et al. (2005). Transcranial direct current stimulation of the unaffected hemisphere in stroke patients. *Neuroreport, 16*(14), 1551–1555.

Fricke, K., Seeber, A. A., Thirugnanasambandam, N., Paulus, W., Nitsche, M. A., & Rothwell, J. C. (2010). Time course of the induction of homeostatic plasticity generated by repeated transcranial direct current stimulation (tDCS) of the human motor cortex. *Journal of Neurophysiology, 105*(3), 1141–1149.

Fridriksson, J., Bonilha, L., Baker, J. M., Moser, D., & Rorden, C. (2010). Activity in preserved left hemisphere regions predicts anomia severity in aphasia. *Cerebral Cortex, 20*(5), 1013–1019.

Fridriksson, J., Moser, D., Ryalls, J., Bonilha, L., Rorden, C., & Baylis, G. (2009). Modulation of frontal lobe speech areas associated with the production and perception of speech movements. *Journal of Speech Language and Hearing Research, 52*(3), 812–819.

Fridriksson, J., Richardson, J. D., Baker, J. M., & Rorden, C. (2011). Transcranial direct current stimulation improves naming reaction time in fluent aphasia: A double-blind, sham-controlled study. *Stroke, 42*(3), 819–821.

Fritsch, B., Reis, J., Martinowich, K., Schambra, H. M., Ji, Y., Cohen, L. G., et al. (2010). Direct current stimulation promotes BDNF-dependent synaptic plasticity: Potential implications for motor learning. *Neuron, 66*(2), 198–204.

Gandiga, P. C., Hummel, F. C., & Cohen, L. G. (2006). Transcranial DC stimulation (tDCS): A tool for double-blind sham-controlled clinical studies in brain stimulation. *Clinical Neurophysiology, 117*(4), 845–850.

Gough, P. M., Nobre, A. C., & Devlin, J. T. (2005). Dissociating linguistic processes in the left inferior frontal cortex with transcranial magnetic stimulation. *Journal of Neuroscience, 25*(35), 8010–8016.

Hamilton, R. H., Chrysikou, E. G., & Coslett, B. (2011). Mechanisms of aphasia recovery after stroke and the role of noninvasive brain stimulation. *Brain and Language, 118*(1–2), 40–50.

Hartwigsen, G., Price, C. J., Baumgaertner, A., Geiss, G., Koehnke, M., Ulmer, S., et al. (2010). The right posterior inferior frontal gyrus contributes to phonological word decisions in the healthy brain: Evidence from dual-site TMS. *Neuropsychologia, 48*(10), 3155–3163.

Hocking, J., McMahon, K. L., & de Zubicaray, G. I. (2009). Semantic context and visual feature effects in object naming: An fMRI study using arterial spin labeling. *Journal of Cognitive Neuroscience, 21*(8), 1571–1583.

Holland, R., & Lambon Ralph, M. A. (2010). The anterior temporal lobe semantic hub is a part of the language neural network: Selective disruption of irregular past tense verbs by rTMS. *Cerebral Cortex, 20*(12), 2771–2775.

Holland, R., Leff, A. P., Josephs, O., Galea, J. M., Desikan, M., Price, C. J., et al. (2011). Speech facilitation by left inferior frontal cortex stimulation. *Current Biology*, *21*(16), 1403–1407.

Iyer, M. B., Mattu, U., Grafman, J., Lomarev, M., Sato, S., & Wassermann, E. M. (2005). Safety and cognitive effect of frontal DC brain polarization in healthy individuals. *Neurology, 64*(5), 872–875.

Jahanshahi, M., & Rothwell, J. (2000). Transcranial magnetic stimulation studies of cognition: An emerging field. *Experimental Brain Research, 131*(1), 1–9.

Kelly, H., Brady, M. C., & Enderby, P. (2010). Speech and language therapy for aphasia following stroke. *Cochrane Database of Systematic Reviews*(5), CD000425.

Kendall, D. L., Rosenbek, J. C., Heilman, K. M., Conway, T., Klenberg, K., Gonzalez Rothi, L. J., et al. (2008). Phoneme-based rehabilitation of anomia in aphasia. *Brain and Language, 105*(1), 1–17.

Kincses, T. Z., Antal, A., Nitsche, M. A., Bartfai, O., & Paulus, W. (2004). Facilitation of probabilistic classification learning by transcranial direct current stimulation of the prefrontal cortex in the human. *Neuropsychologia, 42*(1), 113–117.

Kuo, M. F., Unger, M., Liebetanz, D., Lang, N., Tergau, F., Paulus, W., et al. (2008). Limited impact of homeostatic plasticity on motor learning in humans. *Neuropsychologia, 46*(8), 2122–2128.

Lagopoulos, J., & Degabriele, R. (2008). Feeling the heat: The electrode-skin interface during DCS. *Acta Neuropsychiatry, 20*, 98–100.

Lang, N., Siebner, H. R., Ernst, D., Nitsche, M. A., Paulus, W., Lemon, R. N., et al. (2004). Preconditioning with transcranial direct current stimulation sensitizes the motor cortex to rapid-rate transcranial magnetic stimulation and controls the direction of after-effects. *Biological Psychiatry, 56*(9), 634–639.

Lang, N., Siebner, H. R., Ward, N. S., Lee, L., Nitsche, M. A., Paulus, W., et al. (2005). How does transcranial DC stimulation of the primary motor cortex alter regional neuronal activity in the human brain? *European Journal of Neuroscience, 22*(2), 495–504.

Leff, A., Crinion, J., Scott, S., Turkheimer, F., Howard, D., & Wise, R. (2002). A physiological change in the homotopic cortex following left posterior temporal lobe infarction. *Annals of Neurology, 51*(5), 553–558.

Liebetanz, D., Koch, R., Mayenfels, S., Konig, F., Paulus, W., & Nitsche, M. A. (2009). Safety limits of cathodal transcranial direct current stimulation in rats. *Clinical Neurophysiology, 120*(6), 1161–1167.

Liebetanz, D., Nitsche, M. A., Tergau, F., & Paulus, W. (2002). Pharmacological approach to the mechanisms of transcranial DC-stimulation-induced after-effects of human motor cortex excitability. *Brain, 125*, 2238–2247.

Lindenberg, R., Renga, V., Zhu, L. L., Nair, D., & Schlaug, G. (2010). Bihemispheric brain stimulation facilitates motor recovery in chronic stroke patients. *Neurology, 75*(24), 2176–2184.

Liuzzi, G., Freundlieb, N., Ridder, V., Hoppe, J., Heise, K., Zimerman, M., et al. (2010). The involvement of the left motor cortex in learning of a novel action word lexicon. *Current Biology, 20*(19), 1745–1751.

Loo, C. K., Martin, D. M., Alonzo, A., Gandevia, S., Mitchell, P. B., & Sachdev, P. (2011). Avoiding skin burns with transcranial direct current stimulation: Preliminary considerations. *International Journal of Neuropsychopharmacology, 14*(3), 425–426.

Martin, P. I., Naeser, M. A., Theoret, H., Tormos, J. M., Nicholas, M., Kurland, J., et al. (2004). Transcranial magnetic stimulation as a complementary treatment for aphasia. *Seminars in Speech and Language, 25*(2), 181–191.

Meinzer, M., Djundja, D., Barthel, G., Elbert, T., & Rockstroh, B. (2005). Long-term stability of improved language functions in chronic aphasia after constraint-induced aphasia therapy. *Stroke, 36*(7), 1462–1466.

Meinzer, M., Elbert, T., Wienbruch, C., Djundja, D., Barthel, G., & Rockstroh, B. (2004). Intensive language training enhances brain plasticity in chronic aphasia. *BMC Biology, 2*, 20.

Minhas, P., Bansal, V., Patel, J., Ho, J. S., Diaz, J., Datta, A., et al. (2010). Electrodes for high-definition transcutaneous DC stimulation for applications in drug delivery and electrotherapy, including tDCS. *Journal of Neuroscience Methods, 190*(2), 188–197.

Miniussi, C., Cappa, S. F., Cohen, L. G., Floël, A., Fregni, F., Nitsche, M. A., et al. (2008). Efficacy of repetitive transcranial magnetic stimulation/transcranial direct current stimulation in cognitive neurorehabititation. *Brain Stimulation, 1*(4), 326–336.

Miranda, P. C., Lomarev, M., & Hallett, M. (2006). Modeling the current distribution during transcranial direct current stimulation. *Clinical Neurophysiology, 117*(7), 1623–1629.

Monte-Silva, K., Kuo, M. F., Liebetanz, D., Paulus, W., & Nitsche, M. A. (2010). Shaping the optimal repetition interval for cathodal transcranial direct current stimulation (tDCS). *Journal of Neurophysiology, 103*(4), 1735–1740.

Monti, A., Cogiamanian, F., Marceglia, S., Ferrucci, R., Mameli, F., Mrakic-Sposta, S., et al. (2008). Improved naming after transcranial direct current stimulation in aphasia. *Journal of Neurology Neurosurgery and Psychiatry, 79*(4), 451–453.

Naeser, M. A., Martin, P. I., Baker, E. H., Hodge, S. M., Sczerzenie, S. E., Nicholas, M., et al. (2004). Overt propositional speech in chronic nonfluent aphasia studied with the dynamic susceptibility contrast fMRI method. *NeuroImage, 22*(1), 29–41.

Naeser, M. A., Martin, P. I., Nicholas, M., Baker, E. H., Seekins, H., Kobayashi, M., et al. (2005). Improved picture naming in chronic aphasia after TMS to part of right Broca's area: An open-protocol study. *Brain and Language, 93*(1), 95–105.

Nickels, L. (2002). Therapy for naming disorders: Revisiting, revising, and reviewing. *Aphasiology, 16*, 935–979.

Nitsche, M. A., Cohen, L. G., Wassermann, E. M., Priori, A., Lang, N., Antal, A., et al. (2008). Transcranial direct current stimulation: State of the art 2008. *Brain Stimulation, 1*(3), 206–223.

Nitsche, M. A., Doemkes, S., Karakose, T., Antal, A., Liebetanz, D., Lang, N., et al. (2007). Shaping the effects of transcranial direct current stimulation of the human motor cortex. *Journal of Neurophysiology, 97*(4), 3109–3117.

Nitsche, M. A., Fricke, K., Henschke, U., Schlitterlau, A., Liebetanz, D., Lang, N., et al. (2003). Pharmacological modulation of cortical excitability shifts induced by transcranial direct current stimulation in humans. *Journal of Physiology, 553*, 293–301.

Nitsche, M. A., Grundey, J., Liebetanz, D., Lang, N., Tergau, F., & Paulus, W. (2004). Catecholaminergic consolidation of motor cortical neuroplasticity in humans. *Cerebral Cortex, 14*(11), 1240–1245.

Nitsche, M. A., Liebetanz, D., Antal, A., Lang, N., Tergau, F., & Paulus, W. (2003). Modulation of cortical excitability by weak direct current stimulation – technical, safety and functional aspects. *Supplements to Clinical Neurophysiology, 56*, 255–276.

Nitsche, M. A., Nitsche, M. S., Klein, C. C., Tergau, F., Rothwell, J. C., & Paulus, W. (2003). Level of action of cathodal DC polarisation induced inhibition of the human motor cortex. *Clinical Neurophysiology, 114*(4), 600–604.

Nitsche, M. A., & Paulus, W. (2000). Excitability changes induced in the human motor cortex by weak transcranial direct current stimulation. *Journal of Physiology, 527*(Pt 3), 633–639.

Nitsche, M. A., & Paulus, W. (2001). Sustained excitability elevations induced by transcranial DC motor cortex stimulation in humans. *Neurology, 57*(10), 1899–1901.

Nitsche, M. A., Roth, A., Kuo, M. F., Fischer, A. K., Liebetanz, D., Lang, N., et al. (2007). Timing-dependent modulation of associative plasticity by general network excitability in the human motor cortex. *Journal of Neuroscience, 27*(14), 3807–3812.

Nitsche, M. A., Schauenburg, A., Lang, N., Liebetanz, D., Exner, C., Paulus, W., et al. (2003). Facilitation of implicit motor learning by weak transcranial direct current stimulation of the primary motor cortex in the human. *Journal of Cognitive Neuroscience, 15*(4), 619–626.

Nixon, P., Lazarova, J., Hodinott-Hill, I., Gough, P., & Passingham, R. (2004). The inferior frontal gyrus and phonological processing: An investigation using rTMS. *Journal of Cognitive Neuroscience, 16*(2), 289–300.

Palm, U., Keeser, D., Schiller, C., Fintescu, Z., Nitsche, M., Reisinger, E., et al. (2008). Skin lesions after treatment with transcranial direct current stimulation (tDCS). *Brain Stimulation, 1*(4), 386–387.

Papoutsi, M., de Zwart, J. A., Jansma, J. M., Pickering, M. J., Bednar, J. A., & Horwitz, B. (2009). From phonemes to articulatory codes: An fMRI study of the role of Broca's area in speech production. *Cerebral Cortex, 19*(9), 2156–2165.

Pobric, G., Jefferies, E., & Lambon Ralph, M. A. (2007). Anterior temporal lobes: Mimicking semantic dementia by using rTMS in normal participants. *Proceedings of the National Academy of Sciences, 104*(50), 20137–20141.

Poeck, K., Huber, W., & Willmes, K. (1989). Outcome of intensive language treatment in aphasia. *Journal of Speech and Hearing Disorders, 54*, 471–479.

Poreisz, C., Boros, K., Antal, A., & Paulus, W. (2007). Safety aspects of transcranial direct current stimulation concerning healthy subjects and patients. *Brain Research Bulletin, 72*(4–6), 208–214.

Price, C. J. (2010). The anatomy of language: A review of 100 fMRI studies published in 2009. *Annals of the New York Academy of Sciences, 1191*, 62–88.

Priori, A., Hallett, M., & Rothwell, J. C. (2009). Repetitive transcranial magnetic stimulation or transcranial direct current stimulation? *Brain Stimulation, 2*(4), 241–245.

Pulvermuller, F., Neininger, B., Elbert, T., Mohr, B., Rockstroh, B., Koebbel, P., et al. (2001). Constraint-induced therapy of chronic aphasia after stroke. *Stroke, 32*(7), 1621–1626.

Purpura, D. P., & McMurtry, J. G. (1965). Intracellular activities and evoked potential changes during polarization of motor cortex. *Journal of Neurophysiology, 28*, 166–185.

Reis, J., Schambra, H. M., Cohen, L. G., Buch, E. R., Fritsch, B., Zarahn, E., et al. (2009). Noninvasive cortical stimulation enhances motor skill acquisition over multiple days through an effect on consolidation. *Proceedings of the National Academy of Sciences of the United States of America, 106*(5), 1590–1595.

Rosen, H. J., Petersen, S. E., Linenweber, M. R., Snyder, A. Z., White, D. A., Chapman, L., et al. (2000). Neural correlates of recovery from aphasia after damage to left inferior frontal cortex. *Neurology, 55*(12), 1883–1894.

Ross, L. A., McCoy, D., Wolk, D. A., Coslett, H. B., & Olson, I. R. (2010). Improved proper name recall by electrical stimulation of the anterior temporal lobes. *Neuropsychologia, 48*(12), 3671–3674.

Siebner, H. R., Lang, N., Rizzo, V., Nitsche, M. A., Paulus, W., Lemon, R. N., et al. (2004). Preconditioning of low-frequency repetitive transcranial magnetic stimulation with transcranial direct current stimulation: Evidence for homeostatic plasticity in the human motor cortex. *Journal of Neuroscience, 24*(13), 3379–3385.

Sparing, R., Dafotakis, M., Hesse, M. D., & Fink, G. R. (2007). Enhancing language performance with transcranial direct current stimulation in healthy humans: Implications for rehabilitation and recovery of function after stroke. *Journal of Neurology, 254*, 65–65.

Stagg, C. J., & Nitsche, M. A. (2011). Physiological basis of transcranial direct current stimulation. *Neuroscientist, 17*(1), 37–53.

Stewart, L., Meyer, B., Frith, U., & Rothwell, J. C. (2001). Left posterior BA37 is involved in object recognition: A TMS study. *Neuropsychologia, 39*, 1–6.

Thiel, A., Haupt, W. F., Habedank, B., Winhuisen, L., Herholz, K., Kessler, J., et al. (2005). Neuroimaging-guided rTMS of the left inferior frontal gyrus interferes with repetition priming. *NeuroImage, 25*(3), 815–823.

Vandermeeren, Y., Jamart, J., & Ossemann, M. (2010). Effect of tDCS with an extracephalic reference electrode on cardio-respiratory and autonomic functions. *BMC Neuroscience, 11*, 38.

Vigneau, M., Beaucousin, V., Herve, P. Y., Duffau, H., Crivello, F., Houde, O., et al. (2006). Meta-analyzing left hemisphere language areas: Phonology, semantics, and sentence processing. *NeuroImage, 30*(4), 1414–1432.

Vines, B. W., Cerruti, C., & Schlaug, G. (2008). Dual-hemisphere tDCS facilitates greater improvements for healthy subjects' non-dominant hand compared to uni-hemisphere stimulation. *BMC Neuroscience, 9*, 103.

Vitali, P., Abutalebi, J., Tettamanti, M., Danna, M., Ansaldo, A. I., Perani, D., et al. (2007). Training-induced brain remapping in chronic aphasia: A pilot study. *Neurorehabilitation and Neural Repair, 21*(2), 152–160.

Winhuisen, L., Thiel, A., Schumacher, B., Kessler, J., Rudolf, J., Haupt, W. F., et al. (2005). Role of the contralateral inferior frontal gyrus in recovery of language function in poststroke aphasia: A combined repetitive transcranial magnetic stimulation and positron emission tomography study. *Stroke, 36*(8), 1759–1763.

APHASIOLOGY, 2012, 26 (9), 1192–1217

Epidural cortical stimulation and aphasia therapy

Leora R. Cherney[1,2], Richard L. Harvey[1,2], Edna M. Babbitt[1], Rosalind Hurwitz[1], Rosalind C. Kaye[1], Jaime B. Lee[1], and Steven L. Small[3]

[1]Rehabilitation Institute of Chicago, Chicago, IL, USA
[2]Northwestern University, Feinberg School of Medicine, Chicago, IL, USA
[3]University of California, Irvine, CA, USA

Background: There are several methods of delivering cortical brain stimulation to modulate cortical excitability, and interest in their application as an adjuvant strategy in aphasia rehabilitation after stroke is growing. Epidural cortical stimulation, although more invasive than other methods, permits high-frequency stimulation of high spatial specificity to targeted neuronal populations.
Aims: First we review evidence supporting the use of epidural cortical stimulation for upper limb recovery after focal cortical injury in both animal models and human stroke survivors. These data provide the empirical and theoretical platform underlying the use of epidural cortical stimulation in aphasia. Second, we summarise evidence for the application of epidural cortical stimulation in aphasia. We describe the procedures and primary outcomes of a safety and feasibility study (Cherney, Erickson, & Small, 2010), and provide previously unpublished data regarding secondary behavioural outcomes from that study.
Main Contribution: In a controlled study comparing epidural cortical stimulation plus language treatment (CS/LT) to language treatment alone (LT), eight stroke survivors with nonfluent aphasia received intensive language therapy for 6 weeks. Four of these participants also underwent surgical implantation of an epidural stimulation device, which was activated only during therapy sessions. Behavioural data were collected before treatment, immediately after treatment, and at 6 and 12 weeks following the end of treatment. The effect size for the primary outcome measure, the Western Aphasia Battery Aphasia Quotient, was benchmarked as moderate from baseline to immediately post-treatment, and large from baseline to the 12-week follow-up. Similarly, effect sizes obtained at the 12-week follow-up for the Boston Naming Test, the Communicative Effectiveness Index, and for correct information units on a picture description task were greater than those obtained immediately post treatment. When effect sizes were compared for individual participant pairs on discourse measures of content and rate, effects were typically larger for the investigational participants receiving CS/LT than for the control participants receiving LT alone. These analyses support previous findings regarding therapeutic

Address correspondence to: Leora R. Cherney PhD, Center for Aphasia Research and Treatment, Rehabilitation Institute of Chicago, 345 East Superior Street, Chicago, IL 60611, USA. E-mail: lcherney@ric.org

Preparation of this manuscript was supported by Grant 5R21DC9876 (to LRC) from the National Institute on Deafness and Other Communication Disorders. The authors acknowledge the support of Northstar Neuroscience, who funded this study. The authors note that they have not had any other financial relationship with Northstar Neuroscience, and did not receive any personal compensation from the company.

http://dx.doi.org/10.1080/02687038.2011.603719

efficacy of CS/LT compared to LT, i.e., epidural stimulation of ipsilesional premotor cortex may augment behavioural speech-language therapy, with the largest effects after completion of therapy.
Conclusions: Continued investigation of epidural cortical stimulation in combination with language training in post-stroke aphasia should proceed cautiously. Carefully planned studies that customize procedures to individual profiles are warranted. Information from research on non-invasive methods of CS/LT may also inform future studies of epidural cortical stimulation.

Keywords: Aphasia; Cortical stimulation; Rehabilitation.

Aphasia rehabilitation has focused traditionally on behavioural and environmental interventions. In spite of the extensive literature indicating that individuals with aphasia benefit from such treatment (Albert, 1998; Cherney & Robey, 2008; Holland, Fromm, DeRuyter & Stein, 1996; Robey, 1994, 1998), most patients continue to be left with residual deficits that affect their daily communication as well as their quality of life.

As we acquire new knowledge about aphasia and brain–behaviour relations, novel approaches to treatment are emerging. For example, Small (2002, 2004) has advocated for a biological model of aphasia rehabilitation in which the goal of remediation is to alter brain anatomy and physiology so that language function can be restored. Importantly, the efficacy of biological interventions seems to depend on the presence of concomitant behavioural training. Whereas biological interventions can stimulate the injured brain, repair the physical damage, or make it more susceptible to the effects of training, concomitant behavioural interventions are needed to retrain the new circuitry and/or integrate new or modified circuits with existing (preserved and/or altered) ones. Thus the promise of any biological treatment appears to be as an adjuvant to the behavioural training (Dobkin, 2004).

Facilitating brain plasticity with the direct application of stimulation to the cerebral cortex is a new area of investigation that shows promise for enhancing language recovery in stroke-induced aphasia, most probably when it is combined with intense training. Cortical stimulation approaches are partly based on a model of interhemispheric competition between the injured and the intact hemisphere (Fregni & Pascual-Leone, 2007; Talelli & Rothwell, 2006). According to this model, deficits may result from at least two possible sources: (1) reduced activity or output of the injured hemisphere; and (2) excess inhibition of the injured hemisphere by the relatively preserved contralesional hemisphere. Depending on how it is applied, the cortical stimulation modulates the stroke-induced imbalance of activity between the two cerebral hemispheres. Improvements may occur by either increasing the output of recruited areas of either the injured or opposite hemisphere or decreasing the inhibitory activity of the maladaptive areas of either hemisphere. Support for this hypothesis has come from physiologic and imaging studies showing disinhibition and increased activity of the contralesional hemisphere after stroke in the motor and language domains (Bütefisch, Netz, Wessling, Seitz, & Hömberg, 2003; Rosen et al., 2000).

There are several methods of delivering cortical brain stimulation to modulate cortical excitability (Lefaucher, 2009). These include direct epidural cortical stimulation, repetitive transcranial magnetic stimulation (rTMS), and transcranial direct current stimulation (tDCS), each of which have been studied in animal models with promising results and subsequently applied to the rehabilitation of motor deficits after stroke (Harvey & Nudo, 2007; Talelli & Rothwell, 2006). Application of these methods to language problems after stroke is only now beginning to emerge. Nevertheless, results suggest a potential role for cortical stimulation as an adjuvant strategy in aphasia rehabilitation.

This article focuses on epidural cortical stimulation. Although more invasive than the other methods, it permits high-frequency stimulation of high spatial specificity to targeted neuronal populations, potentially inducing plastic neuronal changes in specific cortical regions of interest. In addition, implanted stimulation may be more clinically useful if tolerated since it avoids the need to re-localise stimulation on a daily basis as is necessary with non-invasive stimulation (Harvey & Nudo, 2007). First we review the evidence supporting the use of epidural cortical stimulation for upper limb recovery after focal cortical injury in both animal models and human stroke survivors. These data provide the empirical and theoretical platform underlying the use of epidural cortical stimulation in aphasia. Second, we summarise evidence related to the application of epidural cortical stimulation in aphasia. Following a description of the procedures and primary outcomes of a safety and feasibility study (Cherney, Erickson, & Small, 2010), we provide previously unpublished data regarding secondary behavioural outcomes from that study. We conclude with comments regarding the future of epidural cortical stimulation as an adjuvant treatment for stroke-induced aphasia.

PRECLINICAL STUDIES OF CORTICAL STIMULATION COMBINED WITH REHABILITATION TRAINING

Table 1 summarises key results from the literature that have demonstrated in animal studies that cortical stimulation (CS) combined with rehabilitation training (RT) enhances motor functional outcomes compared to rehabilitation alone. In a series of early studies, rats were pre-trained on a skilled reaching task before receiving sensorimotor cortex lesions and implantation of chronic subdural electrodes (Adkins-Muir & Jones, 2003; Kleim et al., 2003; Teskey, Flynn, Goertzen, Monfils, & Young, 2003). Following surgery, some of the rats received subdural stimulation of the motor cortex concurrent with repetitive practice in the pre-trained skilled reaching task (CS/RT) while other rats received only the repetitive rehabilitation training (RT) for a period of 10 days. In all the studies performance on the reaching task in rats receiving CS/RT was superior to that of the rats receiving RT. Furthermore, enhanced behavioural function in the CS/RT groups also coincided with neuroanatomical and neurophysiological changes including increased dendritic density (Adkins-Muir & Jones, 2003), enlarged microstimulation-evoked motor maps (Kleim et al., 2003), and enhancement in the polysynaptic component of evoked potentials (Teskey et al., 2003) in ipsilesional cortex compared to those receiving RT alone.

These studies also began to determine optimal stimulation parameters by evaluating different stimulation frequencies and polarities. For example, monopolar stimulation delivers current to the cortex via a single polarity, either cathodal (negative pole) or anodal (positive pole). With monopolar stimulation the current flows into the cortex and exits the body at a remote site. In contrast, bipolar stimulation is delivered with a single electrode where current flows out from one contact on the electrode and returns via another contact on the electrode. The current then flows across the cortex locally underneath the electrode contact area with bipolar stimulation. Kleim et al. (2003) demonstrated that both monopolar and bipolar stimulation induced significant increases in peri-infarct movement representations in comparison to controls. However, monopolar stimulation was more effective at improving motor

TABLE 1
Animal studies of direct cortical stimulation (CS) combined with rehabilitation training (RT) for upper extremity motor recovery

Study	*Animal model*	*Cortical stimulation parameters*	*Rehabilitation training*	*Behavioral outcomes*	*Neuroanatomical / neurophysiological outcomes*
Kleim et al., 2003	Rodent Compared monopolar cathodal, bipolar cathodal, monopolar anodal, and no CS	Subdural 50Hz 1 sec pulse	Single pellet reaching task 20 minutes/day for 10 days	Both monopolar and bipolar CS enhanced motor recovery – monopolar stimulation more effective	Both monopolar and bipolar CS increased area of cortex from which micro stimulation movements could be evoked
Teskey et al., 2003	Rodent Compared frequencies (0, 25, 50, 100, 250, and 500 Hz)	Subdural 0, 25, 50, 100, 250, 500 Hz 3 s pulse 50% MT	Pasta Matrix Task 20 minutes/day for 10 days	CS with frequencies between 50 and 250 Hz more effective Returned to pre-infarct training levels for reaching success	Enhanced evoked potentials and lowering of the MT (25 Hz and above) Larger polysynaptic potentiation between 50 and 500 Hz
Adkins-Muir & Jones, 2003	Rodent Compared frequencies (50 Hz, 250 Hz, and no CS)	Subdural 50 Hz, 250 Hz no CS 3 s pulse 50–70% MT	Montoya staircase – retrieved food pellets placed at variable distances on a "staircase" 20 minutes/day for 10 days	No significant difference in reaching between 250 Hz and no CS 50 Hz group had significantly greater rate of improvement in reaching	50 Hz significant increase in surface density of dendritic processes in perilesion cortex compared to other two groups
Plautz et al., 2003	Nonhuman primate Assessed feasibility of CS/RT in primates	Subdural 50 Hz 50% MT 1 second continuous stimulation – unlimited duration pulse train Monopolar	Unimanual pellet retrieval task requiring skilled use of hand – progressed through training stages in which gradual decrease in the diameter of the wells required increasing finger dexterity Two 35-minute sessions per day for 30 days CS initiated 5 minutes before RT	Significant improvement in motor performance (success, speed, efficiency) of pellet retrieval which persisted for at least 4 months Substantial but incomplete resolution of chronic motor performance deficits	Large scale emergence of new hand representations in peri-infarct motor cortex, notably in cortical tissue underlying the electrode

(*Continued*)

TABLE 1
(Continued)

Study	*Animal model*	*Cortical stimulation parameters*	*Rehabilitation training*	*Behavioral outcomes*	*Neuroanatomical / neurophysiological outcomes*
Plautz & Nudo (2005)	Nonhuman primate Assessed feasibility of CS/RT in primates	Modified stimulus parameters – monopolar cathodal 100 μsec duration 100 Hz 50% MT	Unimanual pellet retrieval task requiring skilled use of hand – progressed through training stages in which gradual decrease in the diameter of the wells required increasing finger dexterity Two 35-minute sessions per day for 30 days CS initiated 5 minutes before RT	Peak recovery level (% recovery to pre-infarct level) was 88% for CS/RT and 43% for RT alone	
Adkins et al., 2006	Rodent Compared anodal versus cathodal stimulation	Epidural 100 Hz monopolar stimulation 50% MT	Single pellet retrieval task 60 trials per day or 15 minutes whichever occurred first for 18 days	Demonstrated efficacy of epidural CS/RT Both anodal and cathodal CS/RT enhanced reaching performance compared to no CS group	Cathodal CS/RT group showed increased neuronal density in perilesion cortex
Adkins et al., 2008	Rodent Compared effect of CS/RT on rats with moderate versus severe retrieval deficits	Epidural 100 Hz monopolar cathodal stimulation 40–50% MT	Single pellet retrieval task 60 trials per day or 15 minutes whichever occurred first for 18 days	CS/RT enhanced recovery of reaching success in the moderately but not severely impaired subgroups.	Both CS/RT groups had increased density of axodendritic synapses compared to no CS and there was a positive correlation between post rehab reaching success and synaptic density
Boychuk et al., 2011	Rodent Compared focal versus distributed CS	Epidural monopolar 1-second, 50-Hz cathodal pulse 50% MT	Single pellet skilled reaching task 15 minutes/day for 12 consecutive days	Only the distributed CS/RT enhanced motor performance with RT	Both the focal and distributed CS/RT promoted motor map reorganisation

CS = cortical stimulation; RT = rehabilitation training; MT = motor threshold.

performance. Teskey et al. (2003) found that rats receiving CS/RT with frequencies between 50 and 250 Hz returned to their pre-infarct training levels, while Adkin-Muir and Jones (2003) found that the greatest rate of improvement in reaching occurred with 50-Hz stimulation as compared to 250-Hz or no stimulation.

More recent studies using a rodent model of focal ischaemia have utilized electrodes placed epidurally, rather subdurally, which more closely mirrors electrode placement in human trials. Importantly, Adkins and colleagues (2006) demonstrated that epidurally delivered cortical electrical stimulation produced results similar to those found with subdurally implanted electrodes. Additionally their study compared anodal and cathodal 100-Hz monopolar cortical stimulation delivered at 50% motor threshold; while both polarities improved forelimb motor movement in rats when combined with rehabilitation training, results suggested that cathodal stimulation may contribute to greater perilesional neuronal density (Adkins et al., 2006).

In a subsequent study, Adkins, Hsu, and Jones (2008) demonstrated that the severity of the behavioural impairment could impact the outcomes of CS/RT. Rats were divided into severely and moderately impaired subgroups based on the initial magnitude of their reaching deficits immediately after infarction. Two weeks later the rats received either 100-Hz cathodal stimulation at 50% of movement thresholds or no stimulation (control) during rehabilitation training on a reaching task. The CS/RT enhanced recovery of reaching success in the moderately but not the severely impaired subgroups. However, both severity groups receiving cortical stimulation had increased density of axodendritic synapses compared to no cortical stimulation, and there was a positive correlation between post-rehabilitation reaching success and density of axodendritic synapses.

Another factor impacting outcomes of CS/RT relates to the distribution of electrical stimulation across the cortex. The animal studies described above have typically used more distributed arrangements of stimulation that include representations of face and proximal forelimb movements. A recent study compared a distributed versus focal arrangement of electrical contacts during CS/RT. Both electrode configurations used four identical contacts; in the distributed configuration they were each placed in the corner of a 2 mm by 2 mm square, whereas in the focal arrangement they were clustered in the centre. The study found that only the distributed form of CS/RT enhanced motor performance in the rodents when combined with rehabilitation, even though both forms of CS/RT promoted motor map reorganization (Boychuk, Adkins, & Kleim, 2011). This finding is important because many of the human studies have delivered the stimulation to a focal region of motor cortex.

Given the promising results from using CS/RT in rodents, its use in humans seemed worth pursuing. However, prior to evaluating the use of such device-assisted cortical stimulation in humans, it was important to evaluate its feasibility in a non-human primate model of focal ischaemia. Adult squirrel monkeys were selected for such a study because their nervous system shares many functional and anatomical complexities with the human nervous system (Plautz et al., 2003; Plautz & Nudo, 2005). Additionally, the motor cortex of the squirrel monkey is located in a relatively unfissured region on the exposed surface of the brain, thereby facilitating detailed functional mapping of motor outputs (Plautz & Nudo, 2005). The monkeys were trained to remove food pellets from wells of decreasing diameter, a task that required increased skilled use of digits. Functional maps of the motor representation of the preferred hand and arm in primary motor cortex were obtained. In the same surgical procedure, an ischaemic infarct was produced, destroying the primary motor cortex hand representation while sparing the surrounding arm representations and premotor hand/arm representations. Several weeks later, a second surgery was performed to remap the motor cortex for lesion verification and to implant a subdural surface electrode over an intact region of peri-infarct motor cortex. Following several months of stabilisation of recovery, the monkeys received 30 days of subthreshold CS/RT. Post-therapy, their behavioural performance was tracked for several months and a third cortical map was derived.

Results showed statistically significant gains in the ability of the monkeys to retrieve the food pellets from the wells with combined CS/RT, although there was not a return to pre-infarct abilities (Plautz et al., 2003). Cortical mapping after the CS/RT showed newly emerged hand representations involving cortex both adjacent to the infarct and a considerable distance from it, with the greatest expansions occurring in the cortex immediately beneath the electrode patch. These results suggested that cortical stimulation can facilitate positive involvement of cortical regions that would not otherwise be involved in recovery (Plautz & Nudo, 2005). In addition to supporting the feasibility of CS/RT to improve motor deficits post-stroke, this study also showed that the intervention does not need to be limited to the immediate post-stroke period; improvements can be obtained when the intervention is provided several months after the infarct. Furthermore, post-therapy performance levels were maintained throughout a follow-up period of at least 4 months (Plautz et al., 2003; Plautz & Nudo, 2005).

CORTICAL STIMULATION COMBINED WITH REHABILITATION TRAINING FOR IMPROVED MOTOR FUNCTION IN HUMANS

Although human trials for regeneration and repair after stroke aim to translate results from animal studies, it is important to note the differences between animal models of stroke and the actual biological manifestations of human stroke (Nudo, 2007). For example, focal artificially induced lesions in animal models usually spare adjacent cortex, whereas in humans lesions are often more diffuse and have lower survival of peri-infarct representations. Additionally, animal models do not have the comorbidities common in adults with stroke, since the experiments are typically undertaken in healthy, young to middle-aged animals, and potential confounds are tightly controlled. In the natural environment clinical stroke is often accompanied by and/or results from complex predisposing conditions such as cardiovascular disease and related obesity, diabetes, hypertension, hypercholesterolaemia, and age, which can change the underlying neural substrate in the brain.

Despite these caveats, much can be learned from animal research, and there has been a progression of human research based on this work evaluating the safety, feasibility, and efficacy of CS/RT for the treatment of upper extremity movement deficits following stroke in humans. For example, with regard to safety, epidural rather than subdural implantation is preferred in human studies because it has been shown to increase the activation threshold and reduce the risk of induced seizure (Bezard et al., 1999). CS/RT studies for upper extremity movement deficits following stroke in humans are summarised in Table 2. Promising results have been evident in case reports (Canavero, Bonicalzi, Intonti, Crasto, & Castellano, 2006; Kim et al., 2008), small Phase 1 pilot studies (Brown, Lutsep, Cramer, & Weinand, 2003; Brown, Lutsep, Weinand, & Cramer, 2006), and larger Phase 2 studies (Huang et al., 2008; Levy et al, 2008). In the Phase 1 study (Brown et al., 2003, 2006), CS was applied at 50 Hz at 50% MT up to a maximum of 6.5 mA, using an implantable epidural electrode device with

TABLE 2
Clinical studies of cortical stimulation (CS) combined with rehabilitation training (RT) for upper extremity motor recovery following stroke

Study	*Number of participants*	*Cortical stimulation*	*Behavioural treatment*	*Behavioural results*	*Safety*
Canavero et al., 2006	1	Extradural CS. Sequential 1-month blocks of anodal or cathodal stimulation for 8 stimulation intervals to left or right motor cortex Each block with different stimulating parameters: low (50Hz) and high (130 Hz) frequency cathodal and anodal stimulation	2 hours a day, 5 days a week of standard neuro-facilitatory physiotherapy	Best benefit during left hemisphere stimulation; no benefit at hand/wrist but improved arm extensions (strength, range of motion, durability) Benefits at both high (130 Hz) and low (50 Hz) frequencies	Transitory head dyaesthesias with left hemisphere stimulation; arm pain which hindered movement and worsened gait with right hemisphere stimulation
Kim et al., 2008	1	Epidural unipolar anodal CS Contralateral motor and premotor cortex 200 μs pulse duration at 50 Hz 1V progressively increased to 5V over 4 weeks	2 hours a day for 4 months of active rehabilitation training	UEFM increased from 35 – 42/66; FIM score for selfcare, mobility, locomotion increased from 82 – 95/126. Improved gait with no assistance from cane or caregiver	No adverse events
Brown et al., 2003	1	Epidural bipolar CS (3x3 array of 3 mm electrodes) Ipsilesional primary motor cortex associated with finger flexion 100 s pulse duration at 50 Hz 4.5mA	3 hours/day 5 days/week 3 weeks	Improved UEFM from 36–46; maintained for 4 weeks	No adverse effects
Brown et al., 2006	8	Epidural bipolar CS (3×3 array of 3 mm electrodes) Ipsilesional primary motor cortex associated with finger and wrist movement 250μs pulse duration at 50 Hz 50% MT; 6.5mA	3 hours/day 5 days/week 3 weeks	29 % improvement in UEFM in CS/RT compared to 9% for RT at week 1; greater decline in RT alone by 12-weeks; at 12-week follow-up, CS/RT statistically better that RT on UEFM ($p = .003$) and hand function score of SIS ($p = .001$)	Complication with externally wired system in two participants

(*Continued*)

TABLE 2
(Continued)

Study	*Number of participants*	*Cortical stimulation*	*Behavioural treatment*	*Behavioural results*	*Safety*
Levy et al., 2008/ Huang et al., 2008	24	Epidural bipolar CS (2 × 3 array of 3 mm electrodes) Fully implanted pulse generator (IPG) Ipsilesional primary motor cortex associated with finger and wrist movement Pulse duration of 250 μs at 50 Hz for 6 weeks or [illegible]01 Hz for 4 weeks depending on protocol 50% MT 6.5 mA	6 weeks for a total of 65 hrs of treatment Protocol 1: 2.5 hours, 5 times/week for 4 weeks; then 2.5 hours, 3 times/week for 2 weeks Protocol 2: 2.5 hours, 3 times/week for 2 weeks; then 2.5 hours, 5 times/week for 4 weeks	Greater improvements in UEFM and AMAT in CS/RT versus RT group; significant difference for UEFM at 6 month follow-up ($p = .042$)	1 acute post-operative seizure unrelated to the device or treatment
Phase III Clinical Trial (Harvey & Winstein, 2009; Plow et al., 2009)	146	Epidural bipolar CS (2 × 3 array of 3 mm electrodes) Fully implanted pulse generator (IPG) Ipsilesional primary motor cortex associated with finger and wrist movement 250μs pulse duration at 50Hz 50% MT 6.5mA	2.5 hours/day 5 days/week for 4 weeks; then 3 days/week for 2 weeks	No significant difference between CS/RT and RT groups in UEFM and AMAT	Not assessed

CS/RT = cortical stimulation with rehabilitation training; RT = rehabilitation training; UEFM = Upper Extremity Fugl-Meyer; AMAT = Arm Motor Ability Test; SIS = Stroke Impact Scale.

a 3 × 3 array of electrodes and an external electrode lead and external pulse generator. Two participants were excluded after implantation due to external electrode lead complications and infection. Therefore, in the following Phase 2 study, the pulse generator was modified and internalised in a subcutaneous pocket in the chest wall, much like a pacemaker, with wire leads tunnelled under the skin to the electrodes. This served to decrease the risks of device-associated adverse events and consequently no infections occurred. This device is also the same device that was used in our feasibility study evaluating epidural CS/RT in individuals with aphasia.

The Phase 2 motor study evaluated two different stimulation frequencies, each administered during a different therapy protocol (Huang et al., 2008). Both protocols lasted for 6 weeks and provided 65 hours of rehabilitation therapy, but with differences in the application of the cortical stimulation. In the first protocol, rehabilitation training was provided to all participants for 2.5 hours, five times a week for 4 weeks, followed by 2.5 hours three times a week for 2 weeks. Investigational participants were given CS during all therapy sessions at a frequency of 50 Hz to primary motor cortex. In the second protocol, rehabilitation therapy was provided to all participants for 2.5 hours three times a week for 2 weeks, followed by 2.5 hours five times a week for 4 weeks. Investigational participants were given CS during the last 4 weeks of therapy at a frequency of 101 Hz. Primary outcome measures were the Upper Extremity Fugl-Meyer (UEFM) and the Arm Motor Ability Test (AMAT). Overall, there was a trend for greater improvement on both outcome measures during the treatment phase, but this was not statistically significant (Huang et al., 2008; Levy et al., 2008). However, a persisting significant treatment effect was seen on the UEFM at the 24-week follow-up such that the CS/RT group maintained gains while the RT control group declined back to baseline (p =.041). This is similar to Brown's (2006) study where patients receiving stimulation maintained a nearly 10 point improvement in UEFM at the 3 month follow-up while the control groups gains declined from 3.9 at 1 week after treatment to a 1.9 point improvement at 12 weeks ($p = .047$).

Based on the design and methodology of the successful Phase 2 study, a pivotal Phase 3 study was implemented (Harvey & Winstein, 2009). The results from 146 participants, released in January 2008, failed to show a significant difference between the CS/RT and RT groups on the UEFM or the AMAT. Given the successful results from animal models and preliminary studies, this disappointing result has led to speculation about why no overall effect was found in the 146 participants. Several such factors have been postulated, including the fMRI methods used to locate the site of stimulation, the distribution of the current to the targeted brain regions, non-customisation of stimulus parameters (e.g., dosage and frequency) to each participant's individual cortical activation and responsiveness to stimulation, and the timing of the cortical stimulation in relation to the behavioural treatment (Plow, Carey, Nudo, & Pascual-Leone, 2009). Unpublished criticism of the study has also suggested that the stimulator may not have been sufficiently powered since only 13 participants had a motor threshold at or below the maximum stimulation of the implanted pulse generator. In addition, cortical atrophy around the lesions may have reduced the power of the stimulation. Given that mechanisms of recovery vary depending on the type and site of lesion, the stage of recovery, and the integrity of descending pathways, epidural cortical stimulation trials may need to carefully individualise both the brain stimulation and the rehabilitation training in order to capture optimal benefits (Plow et al., 2009). These factors are important considerations not only for cortical stimulation trials for motor deficits but also for epidural cortical stimulation trials for post-stroke aphasia.

EPIDURAL CORTICAL STIMULATION AND APHASIA

There are relatively few studies evaluating the application of epidural cortical stimulation combined with behavioural treatment for aphasia. Aphasia is briefly mentioned in a case report examining bilateral extradural motor cortex stimulation in a participant with hemiplegia following a stroke that occurred almost 3 years previously (Canavero et al., 2006). Multiple sequential blocks of stimulation to areas of maximal functional MRI activation were provided in combination with physical therapy. Both low-frequency (50Hz) and high-frequency (130Hz) stimulation, first to the left hemisphere (during four 1-month stimulation intervals) and then to the right hemisphere (during four 3-week stimulus intervals) was administered. The investigators noted that after stimulation to the left hemisphere "speech was more fluid, his train of talk lasted longer". However, no formal comprehensive assessment of language was made. Stimulation to the healthy right hemisphere did not result in any positive changes.

In another case report, unipolar anodal electrodes were implanted epidurally to cover the premotor and motor cortex as well as Broca's area (Kim et al., 2008). The participant was described as having severe dysarthria and severe aphasia resulting from a stroke that occurred 18 months previously. Improvements in motor and language performance were noted after 4 months of treatment involving 50 Hz CS plus rehabilitation training of two hours daily. These included improved "visual response times for picture words stimuli" from 13.7 seconds to 2.97 seconds, and increased articulatory accuracy (from 45% to 59%). With regard to the aphasia, improved recognition of common nouns was noted.

Neither of these case studies provides a detailed description of the aphasia before and after the application of the CS. Neither do they provide information about the behavioural treatment for aphasia that accompanied the CS. Nevertheless, the case reports are valuable in that they are the first published reports of extradural cortical stimulation and aphasia, and they begin to address the safety of CS over extended periods of time. In the first case report there was some indication of transitory head dyaesthesias; in the second case report, no adverse effects were noted.

We conducted the first controlled study comparing epidural CS plus language treatment (CS/LT) to language treatment alone (LT) in a small group of individuals with chronic nonfluent aphasia. While the intent of this phase 1 study was primarily safety and feasibility, preliminary notions regarding the efficacy of CS as an adjuvant treatment for nonfluent aphasia emerged (Cherney et al., 2010). The purpose of this article is to: (1) summarise the procedures and primary outcomes of the safety and feasibility study, elaborating on the details of the behavioural treatment accompanying the CS; and (2) provide previously unpublished data regarding secondary behavioural outcomes that focus on therapeutic efficacy and address the following two questions:

1. Does CS/LT result in language improvements that are greater than those that are achieved by LT alone?
2. Does CS/LT result in language improvements that are maintained, and if so, are they maintained better than those of the LT group?

METHOD

Participants

Four investigational participants who received cortical stimulation plus language therapy (CS/LT) and four control participants who received the identical language therapy (LT) participated in this single-blind randomised control trial.

Participants presented with chronic aphasia (more than 12 months post onset) following a single left-hemisphere ischaemic infarction, confirmed by MRI. Eligibility criteria included the following: nonfluent aphasia (but not global aphasia) with a Western Aphasia Battery (WAB) (Kertesz, 1982) Aphasia Quotient (AQ) score of 20–80; premorbidly right-handed as determined by the Edinburgh Handedness Inventory (Oldfield, 1971); at least a 12th-grade education; English spoken as the primary language; visual acuity no worse than 20/100 corrected in the better eye; and auditory acuity no worse than 30 dB HL at 500, 1000, and 2000 Hz, aided in the better ear. Exclusion criteria were seizure disorders, haemorrhage, or depression as measured by the Center for Epidemiologic Studies Depression Scale (CES-D) (Radloff, 1977; Shinar et al., 1986). In addition, participants who showed no activation of the left lateral premotor cortex with several language-related tasks during fMRI were excluded. All participants provided written informed consent with the approval of the Institutional Review Boards of Northwestern University and the University of Chicago. The study was also approved by the US Food and Drug Administration under an Investigational Device Exemption.

The first four participants who met the inclusion criteria were randomly assigned to the investigational (CS/LT) or control groups (LT). The next four participants were required to be within 10 points on the WAB AQ of one of the already randomised participants. After being matched by aphasia severity, they were assigned to the opposite group. Table 3 shows the primary characteristics of the enrolled participants. The first four eligible randomised participants were participants 001, 002, 005, and 008.

TABLE 3
Participant characteristics

Participant	*Baseline WAB AQ*	*Gender*	*Age*	*Time post-stroke (months)*	*Lesion location*	*Lesion size (% left hemisphere cortical volume)*
Mild-moderate						
002 (CS/LT)	82.25	M	51	194.7	Fronto-insular	5
016 (LT)	79.95	M	42	12.4	Temporal	8
Moderate						
015 (CS/LT)	72.00	M	57	13.3	Fronto-parietal	11
005 (LT)	59.45	F	56	12.7	Fronto-temporal	17
Moderate-severe						
014 (CS/LT)	45.85	M	34	13.7	Temporal	10
001 (LT)	40.0	M	61	29.8	Fronto-insular	7
Severe						
008 (CS/LT)	34.20	F	60	40.8	Parietal	13
012 (LT)	30.75	M	47	13.1	Parieto-temporal	15

For all participants except 001, baseline WAB AQ scores represent the average score of two administrations because more than 30 days had lapsed between baseline assessment and treatment initiation. Subjects are paired for severity based on the initial WAB AQ score, not the averaged baseline score.

Participants are ordered in matched pairs according to the severity of aphasia, as determined by the initial Aphasia Quotient (AQ) of the WAB. Note that the baseline WAB AQ scores in Table 3 represent the average score of two pre-treatment administrations for all participants except 001, because more than 30 days had elapsed between baseline assessment and the initiation of treatment.

Procedures

Participants were assessed at four separate time periods: (1) at entry into the study (baseline); (2) immediately after the 6-week treatment period (post-treatment); (3) 6 weeks following the end of the intervention (6-week follow-up); and 12 weeks following the end of the intervention (12-week follow-up). The speech-language pathologist (SLP) who conducted the assessments was independent of the SLP who provided the treatment and blind to the participant's group assignment; all participants wore complete head coverings to hide possible evidence of recent surgery.

Each assessment period involved three visits on consecutive days for completion of the behavioural tests. At each assessment period participants were evaluated using the WAB. The WAB AQ served as the primary outcome measure, with a 5-point improvement from baseline to post-treatment being considered success (this value exceeds the standard error of the test). If more than 30 days passed between the initial baseline assessment and the beginning of treatment, the primary outcome measure, the WAB AQ, was readministered and the mean of the two WAB AQ scores (baseline and pre-treatment) was used for all subsequent analyses.

Secondary outcome measures included scores on the Boston Naming Test (BNT) (Kaplan, Goodglass, & Weintraub, 2001), caregiver ratings of the Communicative Effectiveness Index (CETI) (Lomas et al., 1989), and several discourse measures. Discourse tasks included descriptions of two composite pictures (Nicholas & Brookshire, 1993). One picture showed a birthday party scene in which a piece of cake had been eaten by a dog, seen hiding under the couch; the other showed an outdoor scene in which two firemen were coming to assist a man who got stuck in a tree while attempting to rescue a cat in the same tree. Participants' responses on the picture description tasks were transcribed and scored for Correct Information Units (CIUs) according to the procedures outlined by Nicholas and Brookshire (1993). CIU analysis provides a reliable standardised rule-based scoring system that evaluates the informativeness of connected speech in adults with aphasia. In addition, a measure of rate of speech in words per minute was obtained. The picture description tasks were completed during each evaluation visit, thereby yielding three scores for CIUs and words/minute at baseline, at post-treatment, and at each of the follow-up periods. Participants were also evaluated with the NIH Stroke Scale (Goldstein, Bertels, & Davis, 1989), the Box and Block Test (Desrosiers, Bravo, Hebert, Dutil, & Mercier, 1994), and selected subtests of the Behavioural Inattention Test (Wilson, Cockburn, & Halligan, 1987).

At baseline and post-treatment, participants underwent task-dependent BOLD functional MRI at 3 Tesla, using T2* gradient echo spiral acquisition with a standard head coil (Noll, Cohen, Meyer, & Schneider, 1995). Tasks performed included (a) observation of a woman in a video producing single syllables "ta", "pa", "tha", and "ka"; (b) verbal repetition of the same syllables produced by the woman in the video; and (c) reading aloud three- to five-word sentences that appeared on the screen. A volumetric T1-weighted scan (120 axial slices, $1.5 \times 0.938 \times 0.938$ mm resolution) was acquired and averaged to provide high-resolution images on which to identify anatomical landmarks and onto which functional activation maps could be superimposed. Detailed fMRI image processing methods have been described previously (Cherney et al., 2010). Participants were considered eligible if there were common areas of activation in the ventral portion of the left precentral gyrus or sulcus (surface anatomy corresponding to Brodmann Area 6lv) between the imitation and observation tasks or between the imitation and oral reading tasks.

Participants randomised to the investigational group (CS/LT) required surgical implantation of the cortical stimulation device. Device implantation was scheduled for approximately 2 weeks after randomisation to permit sufficient time off antithrombotic agents. In the neurosurgical operating room an investigational epidural 2 × 3 grid electrode array, 2.6 × 2.7 cm in total area (Northstar Neuroscience Inc., Seattle, WA, USA) was implanted on the dura over the left ventral precentral gyrus at the site closest to the fMRI activation site using frameless stereotaxic neuronavigation. The electrode lead was tunnelled to a sub-clavicular site and connected to an investigational implanted pulse generator (Northstar Neuroscience). A second surgical procedure was performed to remove the implanted system at the end of therapy, following the post-treatment assessment (see Figure 1).

Intervention

Participants in the investigational group (CS/LT) began treatment 1 week after surgery for placement of the device. Control participants (LT) began treatment

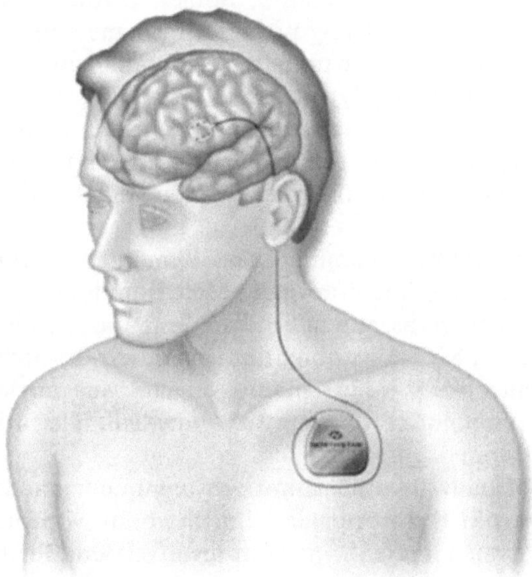

Caution: Investigational device.
Limited by federal (or US) law to investigational use.

Figure 1. Illustration showing the cortical electrode over left ventral precentral gyrus, the electrode lead, and the subclavicular implantable pulse generator (IPG). Note that the lead and IPG were fully internalised. To view this figure in colour, please see the online issue of the journal.

approximately 2–3 weeks after randomisation to parallel the timing of the initiation of treatment for the investigational group.

Both investigational (CS/LT) and control participants (LT) received 3 hours of language therapy per day, 5 days a week, for 6 weeks. Treatment hours were spread throughout the day, allowing frequent breaks for the participants. Investigational participants (CS/LT) also received bipolar cortical stimulation during each therapy session. The stimulator was activated daily prior to the therapy session and deactivated at the end of therapy using a hand-held telemetry device. The target stimulation level was determined prior to the first treatment session and defined as 50% of the language function threshold (i.e., the minimum amount of current required to inhibit language function during a counting task or to elicit movement of the mouth or tongue). If language function was not affected within the programmed parameter limits of the implanted pulse generator then the stimulation level was set to the lesser of the maximum stimulator current or 6.5 mA. One participant (002) received stimulation at 4.75 mA. For all other participants it was set at 6.5 mA. The pulse repetition frequency was 50 Hz and the pulse duration was 250 microseconds (μsec) for all participants.

The language treatment protocol was designed to be (1) representative of what clinicians are doing in clinical practice in that it included practice at each of the phoneme, word, sentence, and discourse levels of language; (2) appropriate for study participants with nonfluent aphasia that spanned a wide range of severities; and (3) clearly and specifically defined to ensure consistency of the intervention over time, between study participants, and across therapists.

The first hour of treatment was provided by a trained SLP and included 15-minute blocks that alternated apraxia drills and rapid cued confrontation naming. The apraxia drills (30 minutes total) emphasised repetitive production of non-meaningful sequences of syllable combinations (Dabul & Bollier, 1976). At the simplest level, participants were required to repetitively produce the same consonant-vowel (C-V) combination (e.g., bah-bah-bah). Over time the C-V combinations were varied (e.g., C_1V_1-C_2V_1; C_1V_1-C_1V_2; or C_1V_1-C_2V_2), increased in length, (e.g., C_1 V_1-C_2V_2-C_3V_3), and increased in complexity to include consonant blends. Participants were required to produce the combinations as fast as they could for 15 seconds at a time, while maintaining accuracy. Integral cueing was provided as needed and gradually decreased as accuracy increased.

In the rapid cued confrontation naming task (30 minutes total) participants were asked to name black-and-white line drawings selected randomly from a core of 200 pictures that included nouns, verbs, and adjectives. Semantic and phonological cueing was provided by the trained SLP according to the hierarchy described by Wambaugh (2003). In one 15-minute block only semantic cueing was provided; in a second 15-minute block only phonological cueing was provided. The order of the cueing blocks was randomised from day to day.

The other 2 hours of daily treatment involved computer practice. Sessions were supervised by the trained SLP who remained in the room with the participant and assisted the participants when needed. One hour involved Oral Reading for Language in Aphasia (Cherney, 2010a, 2010b) in which participants listened to sentences that appeared on the computer screen, pointed to the words as they were said, and then repeatedly attempted to say the sentences, first in unison with the voice on the computer and then independently. Figure 2 shows sample screens from the ORLA programme. The ORLA sentence stimuli allowed practice on a variety of grammatical structures, rather than just one specific grammatical form. There were three levels of

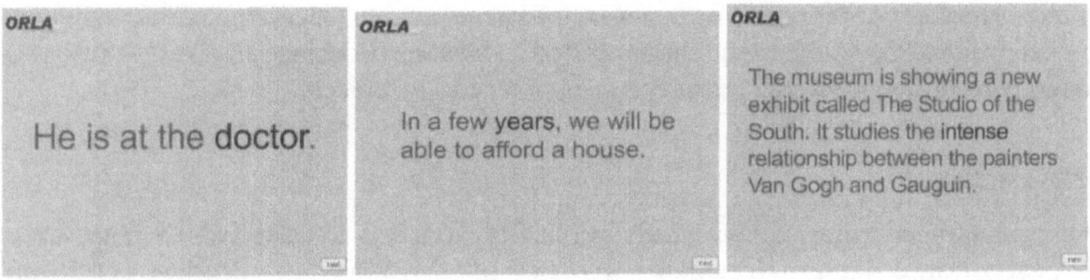

Figure 2. Screen images of the computer-based treatment, Oral Reading for Language in Aphasia (ORLA), showing (a) 3- to 5-word stimulus, (b) 8- to 10-word stimulus, and (c) 15- to 30-word stimulus. To view this figure in colour, please see the online issue of the journal.

difficulty based on length and reading level: level 1 consisted of simple three- to five-word sentences at a first-grade reading level; level 2 consisted of 8–12 words that were either single sentences or two short sentences at a third-grade reading level; level 3 consisted of 15–30 words, divided into two to three sentences, at a sixth-grade reading level. Participants with severe or moderately severe aphasia worked at level 1; those with moderate aphasia worked at level 2, while those with mild-moderate aphasia worked at level 3.

In the third hour participants used AphasiaScripts™, a software program that has been developed to facilitate script training in a realistic conversational context (Cherney, Halper, Cole & Holland, 2008; Lee, Kaye & Cherney, 2009; Mannheim, Halper & Cherney, 2009). In AphasiaScripts an avatar programmed to produce natural speech with correct movements of the speech articulators serves as a virtual therapist or conversational partner. Script practice has three practice modes. First, the participant listened to a pre-recorded script while it appeared on the screen. Second, each sentence or conversation turn was practised repeatedly. Third, the conversation was practised with the virtual therapist while cues were provided depending on the participant's needs (see Figure 3). These cues included seeing the written word, hearing the therapist's voice during choral speaking, and watching oral-motor movements of the virtual therapist. Cues were removed over time so that eventually the participant practised the conversation with the virtual therapist, without cues, as in a real conversation (Cherney et al., 2008). Each week the participants selected two

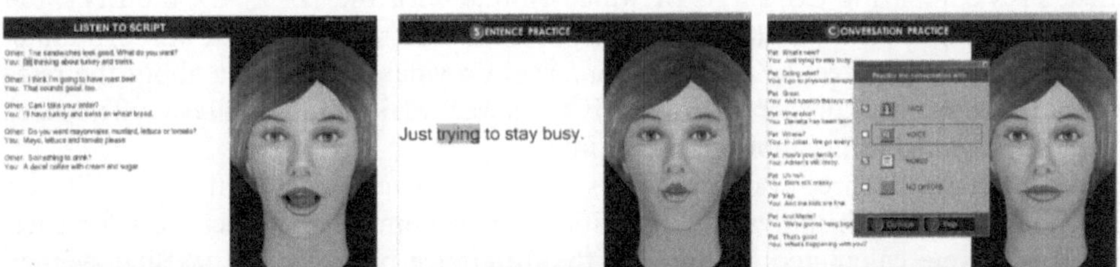

Figure 3. Screens from the AphasiaScripts™ software program showing: (a) listening to the whole script; (b) sentence practice; (c) cues for conversation practice. To view this figure in colour, please see the online issue of the journal.

different conversational scripts from a set of 12 standard scripts. Script topics represented everyday conversational topics such as the weather, deciding on dinner plans, an exercise routine at the gym, shopping for a sweater, ordering in a restaurant, and asking getting-to-know-you questions of a new acquaintance.

Data analysis

The primary endpoint of the study was safety. Safety was assessed by measuring the proportion of study participants with any of the following outcomes: (1) death, (2) medical morbidity, including myocardial infarction, pneumonia, wound infection, or deep venous thrombosis, (3) clinically definite generalised tonic clonic seizure, or (4) decrement in neurological status, defined as a 20% decrease in performance on the neurological, cognitive, and Box and Block testing.

Additional outcome measures assessed aspects of neurobiological change and therapeutic efficacy. Neurobiological change was assessed by measuring activation changes in the syllable imitation task during fMRI in whole brain, each hemisphere, and two regions of interest, the left ventral premotor cortex including pars opercularis of the inferior frontal gyrus (important for speech production and also the site of stimulation on the left) and the left superior temporal gyrus (relevant for comprehension). Therapeutic efficacy was measured by change in language test scores, as described below.

To answer Question 1 regarding language improvements, the change in test scores during the treatment phase (from baseline to post-treatment) for the four participants who received CS/LT was compared with the change in test scores from baseline to post-treatment for the four participants receiving LT alone. These comparisons were made for the WAB AQ, the BNT, the caregiver ratings of the CETI, and the discourse measures of CIUs and words/minute. Given the relatively small number of participants, effect sizes were computed. Effect size measures the magnitude of a treatment effect and, unlike significance testing, is independent of sample size (Cohen, 1988). Cohen's *d* and confidence intervals for the effect size were calculated for the change in test scores from baseline to post-treatment, using the original means and standard deviations of 2 independent groups (Dunlop, Cortina, Vaslow, & Burke, 1996). The effect sizes were benchmarked against Cohen's definition of effect size as follows: small, $d = 0.2$; medium, $d = 0.5$; and large, $d = 0.8$ (Cohen, 1988).

To answer Question 2 regarding maintenance, the changes in test scores from baseline to the 6-week follow-up and from baseline to the 12-week follow-up were compared to the change from baseline to post-treatment within and across groups. Effect sizes comparing CS/LT to LT were computed for the WAB AQ, the BNT, the caregiver ratings of the CETI, and the discourse measures of CIUs and words/minute. Comparison of the effect sizes for each interval provides information about the relative maintenance of skills across groups. If skills were maintained similarly, effect sizes would be expected to be stable across all intervals.

Additionally, the three discourse scores obtained at each assessment period allowed an effect size for each individual participant to be computed. Effect sizes for each participant were calculated by dividing the difference between the baseline average and the post-treatment or follow-up average by the standard deviation of the baseline (Beeson & Robey, 2006). The magnitude of the change from baseline to post-treatment and baseline to follow-up across matched pairs of participants provides an "index of durability" (Beeson & Robey, 2006, p. 167) at different time points following the end of treatment. The benchmarks of 4.0, 7.0, and 10.1 for small, medium and large effect sizes were used to aid interpretation: these benchmarks are based on a meta-analysis for lexical retrieval treatment studies (Robey & Beeson, 2005).

RESULTS

Safety and neurobiological change have been addressed previously (Cherney et al., 2010). In summary, there were no adverse events from either the surgery or the therapy that affected the course of therapy or had a long-term impact on patient well-being. Additionally, neurological, cognitive, and upper extremity motor function remained stable in all participants, as assessed with the NIH Stroke Scale, the Behavioural Inattention Test, and the Box and Blocks Test.

Neurobiologically, for all eight participants combined, decreases in whole brain activation correlated with increases in positive change on the primary outcome measure, the WAB AQ. The inverse correlation between change on the WAB-AQ from pre-treatment to the 12-week follow-up and change in whole brain activation on the syllable imitation task was 0.6159. The ipsilesional left hemisphere showed decreased activation from baseline to post-treatment on all functional MRI tasks, and this decreased more in the investigational group (CS/LT) than in the control group (LT). Different participant pairs did not contribute identically to these values. In general, the participants with mild-moderate aphasia tended to show activation increases, while those with moderate and severe aphasia tended to show activation decreases. These changes differed by brain region and by functional task.

With regard to therapeutic efficacy, Table 4 shows the individual change scores from baseline that were obtained by each participant at each assessment period for the WAB AQ, the Boston Naming Test, and the CETI. It also shows the means and standard deviations of the CIU and words/minute scores that were obtained on the discourse tasks by each participant at each assessment period. In the table participants are ordered by aphasia severity, as determined by the initial WAB-AQ score, to allow for comparisons between matched pairs of investigational and control participants. Table 5 shows the group change scores (means and standard deviations) for the investigational and control groups from baseline for the WAB AQ, the Boston Naming Test, the CETI, and the discourse measures.

Therapeutic efficacy: Group and individual data

Group and individual test data for the WAB AQ, the primary outcome measure, have been reported previously (Cherney et al., 2010). Three of the four investigational participants showed a WAB-AQ change from baseline to post-treatment that was greater than that of the matched control participant (see Table 4). Investigational participants from least impaired to most impaired had increases of 3.45, 7.0, 6.45, and 15.0 points; matched control participants had changes of –0.15, 3.95, 11.9, and 2.65 points. At the 12-week follow-up the most severe participant in the investigational group had an increase of 20.3 points. In comparison, a negative change of –0.5 was shown for the most severe participant in the control group. Although neither the investigational or control participants with mild-moderate aphasia achieved a 5-point

TABLE 4
Change scores from baseline to each assessment period for participants, paired for severity by initial WAB-AQ scores

	Baseline to post-treatment					*Baseline to 6-week follow-up*					*Baseline to 12-week follow-up*				
Participant	*WAB AQ*	*BNT*	*CETI*	*CIUs*	*WPM*	*WAB AQ*	*BNT*	*CETI*	*CIUs*	*WPM*	*WAB AQ*	*BNT*	*CETI*	*CIUs*	*WPM*
Mild-Moderate															
002 (CS/LT)	3.45	−4	35.16	−7.34	12.12	4.25	−1	40.18	20.33	5.62	3.75	2	49.62	27.33	−2.41
016 (LT)	−0.15	−2	−3.44	23.66	12.14	2.35	1	0.94	8.33	22.15	2.45	1	7.31	−3.00	20.08
Moderate															
015 (CS/LT)	7.00	9	16.22	44.66	16.28	2.50	10	19.56	33.33	9.22	7.80	18	15.18	44.66	6.67
005 (LT)	3.95	12	21.80	17.33	−13.94	4.95	12	33.10	14.33	13.73	8.25	11	21.00	25.66	−4.96
Moderate-Severe															
014 (CS/LT)	6.45	−9	MD	5.67	9.80	14.55	1	35.52	14.00	6.24	17.35	−2	37.52	14.33	4.53
001 (LT)	11.90	6	−16.06	15.34	20.31	12.20	11	−3.81	2.34	4.23	LTF	LTF	LTF	LTF	LTF
Severe															
008 (CS/LT)	15.00	10	−0.14	12.00	−1.24	10.60	11	23.25	13.66	−2.41	20.30	15	20.75	15.00	−4.30
012 (LT)	2.65	0	41.31	1.33	−23.28	2.65	0	34.94	6.67	−22.74	−0.50	0	30.81	8.33	−12.63

WAB AQ = Western Aphasia Battery Aphasia Quotient; BNT = Boston Naming Test; CETI = Communicative Effectiveness Index; CIUs = correct information units; WPM = words per minute; MD = missing data; LTF = lost to follow-up.

TABLE 5
Means, SD and effect size (Cohen's *d*) of the change from baseline to post-treatment and follow-up for the investigational group (CS/LT) compared with the control group (LT)

Measure	*Investigational group (CS/LT) mean (SD)*	*Control group (LT) mean (SD)*	*Effect size Cohen's d*	*95% Confidence interval for effect size*	
				Lower	*Upper*
WAB-AQ					
Baseline – Post Tx	7.98 (4.94)	4.59 (5.17)	**0.67**	−0.83	2.00
Baseline – 6 wk f/up	7.98 (5.6)	5.54 (4.6)	0.48	−0.99	1.81
Baseline – 12 wk f/up	12.3 (7.81)	3.55 (4.26)	**1.32**	−0.50	2.72
BNT					
Baseline – Post Tx	1.5 (9.47)	4.0 (6.32)	−0.31	−1.66	1.12
Baseline – 6 wk f/up	5.25 (6.13)	6.0 (6.38)	−0.12	−1.49	1.28
Baseline – 12 wk f/up	8.25 (9.74)	2.0 (6.38)	**0.73**	−0.92	2.15
CETI–CG					
Baseline – Post Tx	17.08 (17.67)	10.89 (25.69)	0.27	−1.27	1.73
Baseline – 6 wk f/up	29.62 (9.8)	16.28 (20.59)	**0.83**	−0.71	2.15
Baseline – 12 wk f/up	30.78 (15.76)	19.62 (11.69)	**0.78**	−0.88	2.19
Discourse: Rate words/minute					
Baseline – Post Tx	9.24 (7.48)	−1.19 (20.7)	**0.67**	−0.83	2.00
Baseline – 6 wk f/up	4.67 (4.97)	4.34 (19.5)	0.02	−1.37	1.41
Baseline – 12 wk f/up	1.12 (5.3)	0.83 (17.1)	0.03	−1.48	1.52
Discourse: Content CIUs					
Baseline – Post Tx	13.8 (22.13)	14.4 (9.42)	−0.04	−1.42	1.35
Baseline – 6 wk f/up	20.3 (9.19)	7.92 (4.97)	**1.68**	−0.10	3.02
Baseline – 12 wk f/up	25.3 (14.21)	10.3 (14.43)	**1.05**	−0.68	2.45

Large and moderate effect sizes are in bold. CS/LT = cortical stimulation with language therapy; LT = language therapy; WAB = Western Aphasia Battery; AQ = Aphasia Quotient; BNT = Boston Naming Test; CETI CG = Communicative Effectiveness Index completed by caregiver; CIUs = correct information units. Post Tx = post-treatment; f/up = follow-up.

change on the WAB-AQ, the investigational participant had greater changes at all time points (Cherney et al., 2010).

Only group data for the CETI have been reported previously. The mean change from baseline to each of the assessment periods was greater for the investigational group than for the control group at all time points (Cherney et al., 2010). Inspection of the individual participant data provided in Table 4 shows that the participant pair with mild-moderate aphasia differed the greatest in CETI change scores. At post-treatment, the CETI change score from baseline was 35.16 points for the investigational participant (002) compared to −3.44 for the control participant (016); at the 12-week follow-up, the CETI change score for the investigational participant was 49.62 compared to only 7.31 for the control participant.

For the BNT, investigational group changes (Table 5) were 1.5, 5.25, and 8.25 points at post-treatment, 6 weeks, and 12 weeks respectively. Respective control group changes were 4.0, 6.0, and 2.0 points. Inspection of individual scores (Table 4) shows that neither of the participants with mild-moderate aphasia made much change from baseline to any time point. Both participants with moderate aphasia improved from baseline to post-treatment and follow-up; the investigational participant (015) improved 18 points while the control participant improved 11 points at the 12-week follow-up. However, although matched for severity on the WAB AQ, there was a large difference in their BNT baseline scores (i.e., 35 for the investigational participant and

7 for the control participant). Conversely, the severe participants with aphasia were evenly matched at baseline on the BNT with a score of zero each. The investigational participant improved 15 points by the 12-week follow-up, while the control participant made no change and remained with a score of zero.

Performance on the picture description tasks yielded different patterns of change for informational content (CIUs) and rate (words/minute) as shown in Table 5. The mean change for the investigational group for words/minute was 9.24, 4.67, and 1.12 compared to –1.19, 4.34, and 0.83 for the control group at post-treatment, 6 weeks, and 12 weeks. Therefore, only at the post-treatment assessment did there appear to be much difference between the two groups. In contrast, for CIUs the mean improvement from baseline to post-treatment was similar for both groups (13.8 for investigational participants and 14.4 for control participants). However, by the 6- and 12-week follow-ups, the mean improvements demonstrated by participants in the investigational group were greater than for the control group (20.3 versus 7.92 at 6 weeks; 25.3 versus 10.3 at 12 weeks).

Therapeutic efficacy: Effect sizes

Regarding language improvements (Question 1), effect sizes for the treatment phase (from baseline to post-treatment) for the four participants who received CS/LT were computed and compared to the effect sizes from baseline to post-treatment for the four participants receiving LT alone. Effect sizes are shown in Table 5. Effect sizes that are positive indicate that the change by the investigational group was larger than the change by the control group. At post-treatment, moderate positive effect sizes are evident for the primary outcome measure, the WAB AQ ($d = 0.67$) and for words/minute ($d = 0.67$).

Regarding maintenance of language improvements (Question 2), effect sizes from baseline to the 6-week follow-up and from baseline to the 12-week follow-up for the CS/LT group were computed and compared to those of the LT group. Large positive effect sizes were obtained for the WAB AQ at the 12-week follow-up and for CIUs at both the 6- and 12-week follow-ups. Moderate positive effect sizes were obtained for the BNT at the 12-week follow-up, and for the CETI at both the 6-week and 12-week follow-ups.

It is interesting to note that, for the WAB AQ, BNT, CETI, and CIU discourse measure, the effect size between baseline and 12 weeks was larger than the effect size between baseline and post-treatment. To interpret the widening difference between the groups, the raw data previously presented in Table 4 were reviewed to determine if the increasing difference in effect sizes over time resulted primarily from continued improvements in the intervention group (CS/LT) or a decline in the control group (LT). While there was some variability, for the most part the increase in effect size at the 12-week follow-up represents continued improvements by the investigational participants following the cessation of treatment.

Tables 6 and 7 include the effect sizes for each individual participant from baseline to post-treatment and follow-up for the measures of CIUs and words/minute. For CIUs, all effect sizes are larger for the investigational than for the control participant within the matched pair except for the baseline to post-treatment period for the participants with mild-moderate aphasia. The large effect size at all assessment periods for the investigational participant with a moderate aphasia (015) is notable. For

TABLE 6
Effect sizes for correct information units (CIUs) computed for each individual participant

	BL to post Tx	*BL to 6-week f/up*	*BL to 12-week f/up*
Mild-moderate			
002 (CS/LT)	−0.64	1.79	2.43
016 (LT)	2.78	0.98	−0.35
Moderate			
015 (CS/LT)	**77.36**	**57.74**	**77.36**
005 (LT)	1.58	1.31	2.34
Moderate-severe			
014 (CS/LT)	2.14	5.29	5.42
001 (LT)	1.66	0.25	Lost to f/up
Severe			
008 (CS/LT)	**7.86**	**8.95**	**9.82**
012 (LT)	1.33	**6.67**	**8.33**

BL = baseline. Effect sizes calculated by dividing the difference between the baseline average and the post-treatment or follow-up average by the standard deviation of the baseline (Beeson & Robey, 2006).

TABLE 7
Effect sizes for word/minute computed for each individual participant

	BL to post Tx	*BL to 6-week f/up*	*BL to 12-week f/up*
Mild-moderate			
002 (CS/LT)	2.69	1.25	−0.53
016 (LT)	2.01	3.66	3.32
Moderate			
015 (CS/LT)	**6.39**	3.62	2.62
005 (LT)	−22.81	22.61	−8.17
Moderate-severe			
014 (CS/LT)	4.04	2.57	1.87
001 (LT)	1.84	0.38	Lost to f/up
Severe			
008 (CS/LT)	−0.13	−0.25	−0.44
012 (LT)	−1.06	−1.04	−0.58

BL = baseline. Effect sizes calculated by dividing the difference between the baseline average and the post-treatment or follow-up average by the standard deviation of the baseline (Beeson & Robey, 2006).

words/minute, effect sizes for individual participants are generally small. It is interesting, though, that some effect sizes are negative indicating that the change from baseline was a decrease in rate rather than an increase in rate. This is seen consistently in both participants with severe aphasia. Additionally, for the control participant with moderate aphasia (005) and the investigational participant with mild-moderate aphasia (002), rate increases or decreases are seen at different assessment periods.

DISCUSSION

This article reports on findings from a safety and feasibility study that evaluated the effects of epidural CS/LT compared to LT in individuals with chronic post-stroke aphasia. Previous reports from this same study indicated that excitatory ipsilesional epidural CS is a potentially safe and feasible adjuvant intervention for individuals with chronic nonfluent aphasia from a single left hemisphere ischaemic infarct that spares ventral premotor cortex (Cherney et al., 2010). In this article we have provided new data about behavioural outcomes that support previous findings regarding therapeutic efficacy of CS/LT compared to LT. The effect size for the primary outcome measure, the WAB AQ, was benchmarked as moderate from baseline to immediately post-treatment and large from baseline to the 12-week follow up. For the secondary outcomes measures, a moderate effect size was obtained for rate of speech on a picture description task immediately post-treatment. At the 12-week follow-up, effect sizes were benchmarked as large for correct information units on the picture description task and moderate for the BNT and the CETI. An analysis of effect sizes for individual participant pairs on the discourse measures revealed effect sizes that were typically larger for the investigational participant receiving CS/LT as compared to the control participant receiving LT alone.

Consistent with findings from the Phase 2 motor study is the persistence of the treatment effect in the CS/LT group, with continued improvements on some measures for at least 3 months post-treatment. The mechanisms of recovery following CS are not well understood. However, the evidence suggests that enhanced neural plasticity with more robust long-term learning and reorganisation of neural circuits plays a role in the improvements in language function associated with the delivery of CS/LT (Hummel et al., 2008). Future research is required to investigate the neurophysiological mechanisms underlying behavioural change, including long-term potentiation (LTP) changes in synaptic efficacy and the role of glutamate-ergic and GABA-ergic intracortical networks as mechanisms of facilitating neuronal plasticity (Hummel et al., 2008).

Limitations of this study have been discussed previously. They include the absence of a sham stimulation arm, the small sample size that precludes significance testing, and differences in participant pairs on variables that potentially may impact therapy outcome such as chronicity, age, lesion location, and lesion size (Cherney et al., 2010). Nevertheless, given these suggestive findings, the next logical steps in the typical progression of clinical research investigating the efficacy of epidural cortical stimulation would include a larger study with more participants, additional behavioural and imaging measures, and a sham stimulation arm. Within a larger study, examination of participant variables that characterise good and poor responders is warranted with the intent of identifying those participants who may be most suitable for epidural CS/LT.

However, interpretation of study results and decisions regarding future research should be made in light of the failed Phase 3 motor study. We still believe that epidural cortical stimulation combined with language therapy holds promise as an adjuvant to behavioural speech and language treatment to improve language outcome. However, continued investigation of epidural CS and language training in post-stroke aphasia should be guided by the same considerations that are given to future research with CS and motor training (Plow et al., 2009). Importantly, a series of carefully planned experimental studies that examine criteria for customising procedures to individual profiles to optimise outcomes may best serve future investigations of epidural CS/LT. Therapeutic parameters that warrant investigation include stimulation montage (monopolar versus bipolar), electrode polarity, local versus diffuse contacts of the electrodes, and the implications of these choices for stimulation within a given region of the cortex. Additionally, information emerging from research on non-invasive methods of cortical stimulation in combination with language treatment, such as stimulation site localisation and stimulus parameters, may inform future studies of epidural CS.

REFERENCES

Adkins, D. L., Campos, P., Quach, D., Borromeo, M., Schallert, K., & Jones, T. A. (2006). Epidural cortical stimulation enhances motor function after sensorimotor cortical infarcts in rats. *Experimental Neurology*, *200*, 356–370.

Adkins, D. L., Hsu, J. E., & Jones, T. A. (2008). Motor cortical stimulation promotes synaptic plasticity and behavioural improvements following sensorimotor cortex lesions. *Experimental Neurology*, *212*, 14–28.

Adkins-Muir, D. L., & Jones, T. A. (2003). Cortical electrical stimulation combined with rehabilitative training: enhanced functional recovery and dendritic plasticity following focal cortical ischaemia in rats. *Neurological Research*, *25*, 780–788.

Albert, M. L. (1998). Treatment of aphasia. *Archives of Neurology*, *55*, 1417–1419.

Beeson, P., & Robey, R. (2006). Evaluating single-subject treatment research: Lessons learned from the aphasia literature. *Neuropsychological Review*, *16*, 161–169.

Bezard, E., Boraud, T., Nguyen, J. P., Velasco, F., Keravel, Y., & Gross, C. (1999). Cortical stimulation and epileptic seizure: A study of the potential risk in primates. *Neurosurgery*, *45*, 346–350.

Boychuk, J. A., Adkins, D. L., & Kleim, J. A. (2011). Distributed versus focal cortical stimulation to enhance motor function and motor map plasticity in a rodent model of ischaemia. *Neurorehabilitation and Neural Repair*, *25*, 88–97.

Brown, J. A., Lutsep, H., Cramer, S. C., & Weinand, M. (2003). Motor cortex stimulation for enhancement of recovery after stroke: case report. *Neurological Research*, *25*(8), 815–818.

Brown, J. A., Lutsep, H. L., Weinand, M., & Cramer, S. C. (2006). Motor cortex stimulation for the enhancement of recovery from stroke: A prospective, multicenter safety study. *Neurosurgery*, *58*, 464–473.

Bütefisch, C. M., Netz, J., Wessling, M., Seitz, R. J., & Hömberg, V. (2003). Remote changes in cortical excitability after stroke. *Brain*, *126*(Pt 2), 470–481.

Canavero, S., Bonicalzi, V., Intonti, S., Crasto, S., & Castellano, G. (2006). Effects of bilateral extradural dortical stimulation for plegic stroke rehabilitation. *Neuromodulation*, *9*(1), 28–33.

Cherney, L. R. (2010a). Oral Reading for Language in Aphasia (ORLA): Impact of aphasia severity on cross-modal outcomes in chronic nonfluent aphasia. *Seminars in Speech-Language Pathology*, *31*, 42–51.

Cherney, L. R. (2010b). Oral Reading for Language in Aphasia (ORLA): Evaluating the efficacy of computer-delivered therapy in chronic nonfluent aphasia. *Topics in Stroke Rehabilitation*, *17*(6), 423–431.

Cherney, L. R., Erickson, R. K., & Small, S. L. (2010). Epidural cortical stimulation as adjunctive treatment for non-fluent aphasia: Preliminary findings. *Journal of Neurology, Neurosurgery, and Psychiatry*, *81*(9), 1014–1021.

Cherney, L. R., Halper, A. S., Holland, A. L. & Cole, R. (2008). Computerized script training for aphasia: Preliminary results. *American Journal of Speech-Language Pathology*, *17*, 19–34.

Cherney, L. R., & Robey, R. R. (2008). Aphasia treatment: Recovery, prognosis, and clinical effectiveness. In R. Chapey (Ed.), *Language intervention strategies in aphasia and related neurogenic communication disorders* (5th ed., pp. 186–202). Philadelphia, PA: Lippincott, Williams & Wilkins.

Cohen, J. (1988). *Statistical power analysis for the behavioural sciences* (2nd ed.). Hillsdale, NJ: Lawrence Erlbaum Associates.

Dabul, B., & Bollier, B. (1976). Therapeutic approaches to apraxia. *Journal of Speech and Hearing Disorders*, *41*, 268–276.

Desrosiers, J., Bravo, G., Hebert, R., Dutil, E., & Mercier, L. (1994). Validation of the Box and Block Test as a measure of dexterity of elderly people: Reliability, validity, and norms studies. *Archives of Physical Medicine & Rehabilitation*, *75*, 751–755.

Dobkin, B. H. (2004). Neurobiology of rehabilitation. *Annals of the New York Academy of Science*, *1038*, 148–170

Dunlop, W. P., Cortina, J. M., Vaslow, J. B., & Burke, M. J. (1996). Meta-analysis of experiments with matched groups or repeated measures designs. *Psychological Methods*, *1*, 170–177.

Feeney, D. M., Gonzalez, A., & Law, W. A. (1982). Amphetamine, haloperidol, and experience interact to affect rate of recovery after motor cortex injury. *Science*, *217*, 855–857.

Fregni, F., & Pascual-Leone, A. (2007) Technology insight: Noninvasive brain stimulation in neurology—perspectives on the therapeutic potential of rTMS and tDCS. *Nature Clinical Practice Neurology*, *3*, 383–393.

Goldstein, L. B., Bertels, C., & Davis, J. N. (1989). Interrater reliability of the NIH stroke scale. *Archives of Neurology*, *46*, 660–662.

Harvey, R. L., & Nudo, R. J. (2007). Cortical brain stimulation: A potential therapeutic agent for upper limb motor recovery following stroke. *Topics in Stroke Rehabilitation*, *14*(6), 54–67.

Harvey, R. L., & Winstein, C. J. (2009). Design for the Everest randomised trial of cortical stimulation and rehabilitation for arm function following stroke. *Neurorehabilitation and Neural Repair*, *23*(1), 32–44.

Holland, A. L., Fromm, D. S., DeRuyter, F., & Stein, M. (1996). Treatment efficacy: Aphasia. *Journal of Speech and Hearing Research*, *39*, S27–S36.

Hummel, F. C., Celnik, P., Pascual-Leone, A., Fregni, F., Byblow, W. D., Buetefisch, C. M., et al. (2008). Controversy: Noninvasive and invasive cortical stimulation show efficacy in treating stroke patients. *Brain Stimulation*, *1*, 370–382.

Huang, M., Harvey, R. L., Stoykov, M. E., Ruland, S., Weinand, M., Lowry, D., et al. (2008). Cortical stimulation for upper limb recovery following ischaemic stroke: A small phase II pilot study of a fully implanted stimulator. *Topics in Stroke Rehabilitation*, *15*(2), 160–172.

Kaplan, E., Goodglass, H., & Weintraub, S. (2001). *The Boston Naming Test*. Philadelphia, PA: Lippincott, Williams & Wilkins.

Kertesz, A. (1982). *The Western Aphasia Battery*. New York, NY: Grune & Stratton.

Kim, H. I., Shin, Y. I., Moon, S. K., Chung, G. H., Lee, M. C., & Kim, H. G. (2008). Unipolar and continuous cortical stimulation to enhance motor and language deficit in patients with chronic stroke: Report of 2 cases. *Surgical Neurology*, *69*(1), 77–80.

Kleim, J. A., Bruneau, R., VandenBerg, P., MacDonald, R., Mulrooney, R., & Pocock, D. (2003). Motor cortex stimulation enhances motor recovery and reduces peri-infarct dysfunction following ischaemic insult. *Neurological Research*, *25*, 789–793.

Lee, J. B., Kaye, R. C., & Cherney, L. R. (2009). Conversational script performance in adults with non-fluent aphasia: Treatment intensity and aphasia severity. *Aphasiology*, *23*(7), 885–897.

Lefaucheur, J-P. (2009). Methods of therapeutic cortical stimulation. *Clinical Neurophysiology*, *39*, 1–14.

Levy, R., Ruland, S., Weinand, M., Lowry, D., Dafer, R., & Bakay, R. (2008). Cortical stimulation for the rehabilitation of patients with hemiparetic stroke: A multicenter feasibility study of safety and efficacy. *Journal of Neurosurgery*, *108*, 707–714.

Lomas, J., Pickard, L., Bester, S., Elbard, H., Finlayson, A., & Zoghaib, C. (1989). The Communicative Effectiveness Index: Development and psychometric evaluation of a functional communication measure for adult aphasia. *Journal of Speech and Hearing Disorders*, *54*, 113–124.

Mannheim, L., Halper, A. S., & Cherney, L. R. (2009). Patient-reported changes in communication after computer based script training for aphasia. *Archives of Physical Medicine and Rehabilitation*, *90*(4), 623–627.

Nicholas, L. E., & Brookshire, R. H. (1993). A system for quantifying the informativeness and efficiency of connected speech of adults with aphasia. *Journal of Speech and Hearing Research*, *36*, 338–350.

Noll, D. C., Cohen, J. D., Meyer, C. H., & Schneider, W. (1995). Spiral K-space MR imaging of cortical activation. *Journal of Magnetic Resonance Imaging*, *5*(1), 49–56.

Nudo, R. J. (2007). Postinfarct cortical plasticity and behavioral recovery. *Stroke*, *38*, 840–845.

Oldfield, R. C. (1971). The assessment and analysis of handedness: The Edinburgh Inventory. *Neuropsychologia*, *9*(1), 97–113.

Plautz, E. J., Barbay, S., Frost, S. B., Friel, K. M., Dancause, N., Zoubina, E. V., et al. (2003). Post-infarct cortical plasticity and behavioural recovery using concurrent cortical stimulation and rehabilitative training: A feasibility study in primates. *Neurological Research*, *25*, 801–810.

Plautz, E. J., & Nudo, R. J. (2005). *Neural plasticity and functional recovery following cortical ischaemic injury*. Proceedings of the IEEE, Engineering in Medicine and Biology 27th Annual Conference, Shanghai, China.

Plow, E. B., Carey, J. R., Nudo, R. J., & Pascual-Leone, A. (2009). Invasive cortical stimulation to promote recovery of function after stroke: A critical appraisal. *Stroke*, *40*, 1926–1931.

Radloff, L. S. (1977). The CES-D Scale: A self-report depression scale for research in the general population. *Applied Psychological Measurement*, *3*, 385–401.

Robey, R. R. (1994). The efficacy of treatment for aphasic persons: A meta-analysis. *Brain and Language*, *47*, 582–608.

Robey, R. R. (1998). A meta-analysis of clinical outcomes in the treatment of aphasia. *Journal of Speech Language Hearing Research*, *41*, 172–187.

Robey, R. R., & Beeson, P. M. (2005). Aphasia treatment: Examining the evidence. Presentation at the American Speech Language Hearing Association Annual Convention, San Diego, CA (November, 2005).

Rosen, H. J., Petersen, S. E., Linenweber, M. R., Snyder, A. Z., White, D. A., Chapman, L., et al. (2000). Neural correlates of recovery from aphasia after damage to left inferior frontal cortex. *Neurology, 55*(12), 1883–1894.

Shinar, D., Gross, C. R., Price, T. R., Banko, M., Bolduc, P. L., & Robinson, R. G. (1986). Screening for depression in stroke patients: The reliability and validity of the Center for Epidemiologic Studies Depression Scale. *Stroke, 17*, 241–245.

Small, S. L. (2002). Biological approaches to the treatment of aphasia. In A. Hillis (Ed.), *Handbook on adult language disorders: Integrating cognitive neuropsychology, neurology, and rehabilitation* (pp. 397–411). Philadelphia, PA: Psychology Press.

Small, S. L. (2004). The biology of aphasia rehabilitation: Pharmacological perspectives. *Aphasiology, 18*(5/6/7), 473–492.

Talelli, P., & Rothwell, J. (2006). Does brain stimulation after stroke have a future? *Current Opinions in Neurology, 19*, 543–550.

Teskey, G. C., Flynn, C., Goertzen, C. D., Monfils, M. H., & Young, N. A. (2003). Cortical stimulation improves skilled forelimb use following a focal ischaemic infarct in the rat. *Neurological Research, 25*, 794–800.

Wambaugh, J. L. (2003). A comparison of the relative effects of phonologic and semantic cuing treatments. *Aphasiology, 17*, 433–441.

Wilson, B., Cockburn, J., & Halligan, P. (1987). Development of a behavioural test of visuospatial neglect. *Archives of Physical Medicine & Rehabilitation, 68*, 98–102.

THE 43rd ANNUAL CLINICAL APHASIOLOGY CONFERENCE

May 28th – June 2nd 2013

Tucson, Arizona, USA

CALL FOR PAPERS

The Clinical Aphasiology Conference (CAC) is an annual forum for clinicians and researchers engaged in the study and clinical management of persons with acquired neurologic language disorders. At CAC, participants present their recent research and engage in extensive discussions with colleagues. To develop an informal atmosphere conducive to the free exchange of ideas, CAC attendance is limited to approximately 100 people. The 2013 Conference Chairperson is Leanne Togher; the Program Chairperson is Monica Strauss Hough.

To Attend the Clinical Aphasiology Conference

If you wish to attend the 2013 CAC, you must submit a summary of an original paper or poster no later than Monday, January 21st, 2013. Two authors from each accepted proposal will be invited to attend the conference. As space permits, first authors of proposals that are not accepted for presentation also will be invited to attend. A number of student fellowships are available on a competitive basis to students who have earned authorship on a paper submitted to CAC.

Scope of Papers and Posters

APHASIA APRAXIA OF SPEECH RIGHT HEMISPHERE COMMUNICATION

COGNITIVE-COMMUNICATION DISORDERS FOLLOWING TRAUMATIC BRAIN INJURY

COMMUNICATION IMPAIRMENTS RELATED TO DEMENTIA

COGNITIVE-LINGUISTIC PERFORMANCE IN ELDERLY ADULTS

FOR DETAILED INFORMATION ABOUT CAC 2013 AND THE CALL FOR PAPERS SEE http://www.regonline.com/clinicalaphasiology

For general information about the Clinical Aphasiology Conference, see: http://clinicalaphasiology.org.

Please send queries to Monica Strauss Hough, PhD, 2013 CAC Program Chair at mshough@fiu.edu

Submitting a paper to APHASIOLOGY

Aphasiology is concerned with all aspects of language impairment and related disorders resulting from brain damage. Submissions are encouraged on theoretical, empirical and clinical topics from any disciplinary perspective, and submissions which involve cross disciplinary study are particularly welcome. *Aphasiology* will publish experimental and clinical research papers, reviews, theoretical notes, comments and critiques. Research reports can be group studies, single-case studies or surveys, on psychological, linguistic, medical and social aspects of aphasia. Submissions and ideas for the Review Articles and the Forum are welcome, and interdisciplinary peer commentary is encouraged. *Aphasiology* articles have a maximum limit of 7,500 words. This 7,500 is to include main text and references only. It excludes title, author's contact details, abstract, figures, tables, captions, and footnotes.

Submissions and books for, or offers to, review should be sent to an Editor, address on inside front cover.

Structured Abstracts
Authors submitting papers should note that the journal uses Structured Abstracts. There is good evidence that Structured Abstracts are clearer for readers and facilitate better appropriate indexing and citation of papers.

The essential features of the Structured Abstract are given below. Note in particular that any clinical implications should be clearly stated.

Abstract (between 150–400 words)
Background: Describe the background to the study.
Aims: State the aims and objectives of the study including any clear research questions or hypotheses.
Methods & Procedures: To include: outline of the methodology and design of experiments; materials employed and subject/participant numbers with basic relevant demographic information; nature of the analyses performed.
Outcomes & Results: Outline the important and relevant results of the analyses.
Conclusions: State the basic conclusions and implications of the study. State, clearly and usefully, if there are implications for management, treatment or service delivery.

Review Abstract
Background: Outline the background to the review.
Aims: State the primary objective of the paper, the reasons behind your critical review and analyses of the literature, and your approach and methods if relevant.
Main Contribution: Give the main outcomes of the paper and results of analyses; and any implications for future research and for management, treatment or service delivery.
Conclusions: State your main conclusions.
All submissions should be made online at *Aphasiology*'s Manuscript Central site (http://mc.manuscriptcentral.com/paph).

Papers are accepted for consideration on condition that you will accept and warrant the following conditions:

1. You will transfer copyright to Psychology Press, should the work be accepted for publication.
2. The work is your original work, and cannot be construed as plagiarising any other published work.
3. You own the copyright in the work.
4. You are empowered by your fellow author(s) to make a submission to this journal, and to make any agreement relating to the work.
5. Your work has not previously been published in the English language.
6. Your work is not under consideration for publication elsewhere, in any form.
7. You have secured the necessary permission in writing from the appropriate authorities for the reproduction in your work of any text, illustration, or other material which is reproduced or derived from a copyrighted source.
8. You have agreed with your fellow author(s) the order of names for publication of the work.
9. You warrant that the work does not include content that is abusive, defamatory, libellous, obscene, fraudulent, or in violation of applicable laws.

If it is found acceptable for publication, you shall retain the right to use the substance of the above work in future works, on condition that you acknowledge its prior publication in the journal, and the publishers Psychology Press.

Free article access
As corresponding author, you will receive free access to your article on Taylor & Francis Online. You will be given access to the *My authored works* section of Taylor & Francis Online, which shows you all your published articles. You can easily view, read, and download your published articles from there. In addition, if someone has cited your article, you will be able to see this information. We are committed to promoting and increasing the visibility of your article and have provided this guidance <http://journalauthors.tandf.co.uk/beyondpublication/promotearticle.asp> on how you can help.